LEARNING SKILLS

An Experiential Guide for Nurses

2nd Edition

PHILIP BURNARD
MSc RMN RGN Dip N Cert Ed RNT

*Lecturer in Nursing Studies,
University of Wales College of Medicine
Cardiff, Wales.*

*Honorary Lecturer in Nursing Studies
Institute for Higher Professional Education,
Hogeschool Midden Nederland,
Utrecht, Netherlands*

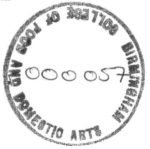

Heinemann Nursing: Oxford

Heinemann Nursing
An imprint of Heinemann Professional Publishing Ltd
Halley Court, Jordan HIll, Oxford OX2 8EJ

OXFORD   LONDON   SINGAPORE
NAIROBI   IBADAN   KINGSTON

First published 1985
Reprinted 1986, 1988
Second edition published 1990

British Library Cataloguing in Publication Data
Burnard, Philip
   Learning human skills.–2nd. ed.
   1. Nurses. Professional education. Curriculum subjects.
   Social skills. Teaching methods: Experiential learning
   I. Title
   610.730711

   ISBN 0-433-00432-0

Typeset from authors' disk by BP Integraphics, Bath and printed in
Great Britain by Biddles Ltd, Guildford and Kings Lynn

For Sally, Aaron and Rebecca and also for John Heron

CONTENTS

PREFACE

We not only live and work with other people. We also live and work with ourselves. The theme of this book is that if we can get to know ourselves better we are likely to be of much greater help to others. The first part of the book explores the notions of self and self-awareness. It also describes and investigates the concept of experiential learning: the means of learning through experience. The second half of the book offers concrete examples of how to put the first part into practice. It offers a discussion of the interpersonal skills involved in one-to-one counselling and in group work and suggests a range of exercises that can help in the development of these. Sample programmes of how to run counselling, group and self-awareness workshops are also offered.

In this second edition, I have aimed at expanding the text to incorporate new developments in the field of experiential learning in nursing and I have incorporated some research into the text. I have added more activities and tried to make more explicit the processes of running experiential learning groups. I hope, more than anything, that the book will be *practical*. It is aimed at a variety of groups of people from student nurses who may want to use it as a means of making sense of their experience, to nurse educators and trainers who may find it useful as a sourcebook. Nurse managers and nurses working in the clinical field may also find it helpful in sparking off ideas about how to run groups and how to learn counselling skills. I know, also, that it has proved useful in the training of health professionals other than nurses.

I have included a number of short case studies, drawn from my research into experiential learning. It is hoped that they clarify some of the issues under discussion: particularly how to put into practice some of the theory. A bibliography of further reading has also been added.

I enjoyed writing and rewriting this book. I would welcome any comments of suggestions that you may have about it.

Philip Burnard,
Caerphilly,
South Wales.

PART ONE

Self-awareness and Experiential Learning

1

The Self and Self-awareness

> The question of identity opens up in two directions.
> On the one hand there is the necessity for a strong
> and clear sense of one's own individuality, one's ego,
> independence, and distinctness in relation to others.
> But with it there comes also the realisation of the
> individuality of others, and of an existence in others
> that is both separate from us and intimately
> connected with us. (Progoff 1985)

We all need self-awareness. It is the basic prerequisite of all skilful nursing. But why? This chapter lays out some of the reasons why all nurses need to develop self-awareness in order to enhance their nursing care. It also explores the complicated issue of what it means to talk about 'self'.

Philosophers and the self

What do we mean when we talk about 'the self'? Of what is the self composed? Is it part of our physical make up? Is it something spiritual? Is it something separate to the body and if so, what is its *relationship* to the body? Questions like these have interested philosophers and theologians for centuries. These days psychologists tackle the problem. The existential school of philosophy discussed the issue under the heading of 'ontology': the study of being. To talk of the self, in this context, is to talk of something more than just bodily existence. It is to describe the fact of being a conscious, knowing human being. Sartre (1956) has written of 'authenticity'; the state of true and honest presentation of being. The authentic person, for Sartre, is one who consistently acts in accordance with their own values, wishes and feelings, making no attempt to play act or to adopt a facade. That person also recognizes the 'being' of others and realizes that when with someone else, that other person is also a conscious, valuing, thinking being. Martin Buber (1958) calls this the I-Thou relationship: the meeting of two people who respect each other's humanity. He contrasts the I-Thou relationship with the I-It relationship. The person who adopts an I-It stance in relationship with another person does not recognize the other as a human being (with all that involves) but treats the other as an 'object'.

R.D. Laing developed these notions and wrote of the 'true' and 'false' self (Laing 1959). The true self is the inner, private sense of self. The false self is the outer, often pretending sense of self. According to Laing, the true self often watches what the false self is doing and a sense of contempt is experienced. The false self is often compliant to the demands of others and can be artificial and insincere. In Sartre's terms, the false self acts inauthentically. The person who has a strong sense of the true self, who is able to act authentically and genuinely is deemed by Laing to have ontological security: security and strength of being. Such security can enable the person to feel able to act rather than to feel acted upon, to make decisions and to feel generally more autonomous. Such a person is also likely to respect the autonomy and self-respect of others. This is not to be confused with selfishness or arrogance—quite the opposite. The ontologically secure person is all too aware of human frailty but, despite it, remains determined to act in a genuine and honest way. It takes courage to be this way.

We can see examples of Sartre's and Laing's ideas in nursing practice. When I was a patient in hospital, I became very aware of how some nurses adopt the 'role of the nurse' as they enter a ward: they suddenly become 'someone else'. It is as though they leave part of themselves behind as they go to work. They have one 'self' for their patients and another for friends and colleagues. If we notice that we are 'acting the role of the nurse' in talking with patients, rather than being outselves, then we are acting in an inauthentic manner. This is not a plea for lack of professionalism but just to note that there is a world of difference between nurses who are open, genuine and sincere and ones who adopt a professional façade, an artificial manner and who fool no one— neither themself, their colleagues and least of all their patients. Nurses who begin to develop self-awareness can monitor their own behaviour and note tendencies towards adopting such a veneer.

Psychologists and the self

Psychologists have approached the concept of self from a variety of points of view. Some have attempted to analyse the factors that go to make up the self rather in the way that a cook might try to discover the ingredients that have gone into a cake. Others have argued that there are certain consistent aspects of the self that determine to some extent the way in which we conduct our lives. Psychoanalytical theory for instance, argues that early childhood experiences profoundly affect and shape the self, determining how, as adults, we react to the world about us. Childhood experiences in this model, lay foundations of the self which may be modified through the process of growing up but which, nevertheless, stay with us throughout our lives. Such a view is *deterministic*: our present sense of self is determined by earlier life experiences.

Other psychologists acknowledge problems with reductionist theories—theories that attempt to analyse the self into parts. They prefer to view the self from a holistic or gestalt perspective. The gestalt approach argues that the whole or totality of the self is always something different to and larger than, the sum of the aspects that make it up. Just as we cannot discover the true nature of a piece of music by examining the piece note by note, neither can we understand the self, completely, by analysing it into separate aspects.

Still other psychologist's take the view that the sense of self is dynamic and every changing. There is no core or *real* self. What we call *self* at any given time is that moments set of beliefs, values and ideas that colour our view of the world. George Kelly (1955) suggested the metaphor of 'goggles'; we all look at the world, at ourselves and at others, through different goggles that are coloured by our beliefs, values and experiences up to that moment. As our beliefs, values and experiences change, so to, do the tints of our 'goggles'. Thus, for Kelly, the person is in a constant state of flux—developing, growing and changing as he/she encounters life. For Kelly, we *are* what we perceive ourselves to be or as the novelist, Kurt Vonnegut put it, 'We are what we pretend to be' (Vonnegut, 1968). Kelly also noted that we *are* what *other people* perceive us to be. We do not exist in isolation. What we are and who we are depends upon the other people with whom we live, work and relate. Our sense of self often depends upon the reports about us that we receive from others. In this sense, other people are telling us who we are. As nurses we rely on patients, colleagues, educators and managers offering us both positive and negative feedback. We absorb such feedback and incorporate the bits that we need to into our sense of self. Sometimes reports from others seem important, at other times they seem less necessary. In the exercises in part two of this book, this notion of receiving feedback from others is explored as part of a self-awareness programme.

Aspects of the self

The self is a complicated concept. It is worth emphasizing the word *concept*. The self is not a *thing* in the way that our liver or lungs are 'things'. The notion of self is an abstraction, a way of talking. It is a shorthand for that part of us that is concerned with thinking, feeling, valuing, evaluating and so forth. While, in one sense, the mind and body are one, in another, they are different if only in that the body is a *thing*, an object in the world, whilst the 'self' is a construct. To talk about the 'mind and body' is tricky for it suggests that two similar sorts of items are under discussion. One way of clarifying what is contained within the concept of self is to consider the notion of *personhood*. If we can identify those basic criteria that distinguish persons from other sorts of things we may be clearer about what it means to talk about the self. Bannister and Fransella maintain that such a list of criteria for personhood will include at least the following items. It is argued that you consider yourself a person because you;

- believe in your own separateness from others; you rely on the privacy of your own consciousness
- entertain a notion of the integrality or completeness of your experience, and that all your experiences are relatable because you are the experiencer
- entertain a notion of your own continuity over time; you possess your own biography and live in relation to it
- entertain a notion of the causality of your actions; you have purposes, your intentions, you accept a partial responsibility for the effects of what you do
- entertain a notion of other persons by analogy with yourself; you assume a comparability of subjective experience (Bannister and Fransella 1986).

These criteria bring together many of the ideas discussed above. They acknowledge the person's uniqueness and difference to others; they acknowledge the person's continuity with the past and they acknowledge their relatedness with other people. We do not exist in isolation; we can assume that we share the planet with other people who are, to a greater or lesser degree, like us.

Another way of considering the concept of self is to consider *aspects* of it. While, as we have noted, all the aspects tend to work together in harmony (we hope!), they are most easily discussed as parts. John Rowan has taken something of a similar approach in his discussion of 'subpersonalities' (Rowan 1989) which he describes as semi-permanent, semi-autonomous regions of the personality. The analysis offered here is not an exhaustive one of all aspects of the self (as we noted above, what *individuals* call 'self' will vary from person to person). It is offered as a means of highlighting the complex and multifaceted nature of the concept of self. The aspects of self discussed here are;

1. the physical aspect,
2. the spiritual aspect,
3. the darker aspect,
4. the social aspect.

The physical aspect of self

The physical aspect of the self is the bodily, 'felt' sense of self; it includes the totality of our physical bodies. In fact one way of considering the self is to consider sense as being a product of the body: bodies generate 'selves'. After all, the chemistry that goes to make up our bodies is also the chemistry that produces our 'mind', that it turn, produces our sense of self. The physical aspect of self covers all those things such as how we feel about our bodies, our sense of body image, our appreciation of how fat or thin we are and so on. It is notable (rather painfully, sometimes) that *our own* perception of our body is not necessarily the perception that others have.

The spiritual aspect of self

Human beings seem to have an inbuilt need to invest what they do with meaning. The spiritual dimension of the person may best be described as that part that is concerned with the generation of meaning. For some, that sense of meaning will be framed in religious terms but it may not be. For others, meaning may be discovered through philosophy, politics, psychology, sociology and so on.

People's meaning systems vary both in their overall structure and in their content. One thing seems certain, it is meaning (or the search for it) that motivates us for much of the time. Jung (1978) described this question for meaning as 'individuation'; the search for the self which was both lonely and difficult. He suggested that one possible outcome of individuation was the realization of both the individual nature of the person and also the person's unity with all other persons. In this context, Carl Rogers noted that 'what is most personal is most general' (Rogers 1967); there is a certain universality about the business of being human.

The darker aspect of self

There is an aspect in all of us that tends towards the negative. While it has become popular to discuss the positive aspects of the self and to theorize about Maslow's (1972) notion of self-actualization—the realization of our full potential—there seems little doubt that we also have a darker side. Jung described this darker side as 'The Shadow' and wrote about it thus:

> Unfortunately there is no doubt that man is, as a whole, less good than he imagines himself or wants to be. Everyone carries a shadow, and the less it is embodied in the individual's conscious life, the blacker and denser it is ...' (Jung, 1938).

Jung suggests that if we want truly to become self-aware, we must be prepared to explore that darker side to our personalities. No easy task! Most of us would rather deny that side of ourselves or rationalize our negative thoughts and behaviour. Sometimes, however, we give ourselves away—particularly through the use of the mental mechanism known as *projection*. With projection we label others with qualities that are our own but of which we are unaware. Often we notice the bad bits of other people while studiously avoiding our own bad bits. This is very evident when we begin to get judgemental and pious about other people. Whilst the shadow may not be the easiest aspect of ourselves to face, it is likely that acknowledging the darker side can help us to accept the darker side of others.

The social aspect of self

The social self is that aspect of the person which is shared with others. It is our presentation of self in various social situations. Consider, for example, you at work. Consider, then, you at home. Finally, consider you with your closest friend. You may well find that you are considering almost three different people! We tend to modify aspects of our presentation of self according to the people we are with and according to what we anticipate will be their expectations of us. This social self then, is closely linked to the self-as-defined-by-others. We do not live as isolated beings. We are dependent upon others to tell use about ourselves. More than that, we *are* different for other people. Consider how the following people view you: your mother, your teacher, your boy- or girlfriend. In each case, those people will see a different 'you' and yet they are all looking at the same person.

Models of the self

These then are aspects of the self—a few aspects amongst many. What is required now is a model that helps to bring all of these aspects into perspective. In its simplest form, the self as a totality can be seen as being made up of three areas or focuses of interest. Figure 1.1 shows these three domains; thoughts, feelings and behaviour.

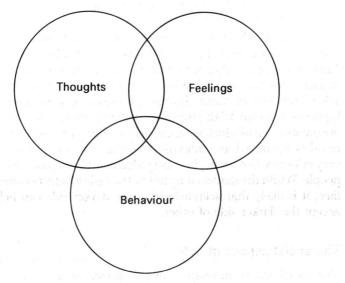

Fig. 1.1 *A simple model of the self*

Each is intimately linked with the other. By thoughts it is meant the processes of ideas, puzzlement and problem-solving that make up our mental life. By feelings it is meant the emotional aspects of our being; happiness, grief, love, anger, joy etc. Behaviour refers to any action that we carry out, to the spoken word and to what is usually called non-verbal behaviour; eye contact, facial expressions, gestures, proximity to others. All three aspects of self in this simple model of self, overlap. We cannot think without in some way feeling. Feelings lead to changes in behaviour even though these are sometimes very small changes. For example, if someone is in the room with you now, just notice them and observe how you can tell that they are thinking or feeling. You will observe changes in eye contact, facial expression or perhaps arm or leg movements. Their behaviour changes again if they notice that you are looking at them; their thinking and feeling changes as they become aware of you and their behaviour changes as a result. We cannot *stop* behaving any more than we can stop communicating.

This interrelatedness of thinking, feeling and behaviour is noticeable from any other starting point. If we ponder for a moment on how we are feeling, such pondering involves thinking and, in turn, a change in behaviour. Here, then, is a starting point for approaching the study of the self. We may study each of the domains and come to know something more about ourselves. As we study each domain and appreciate the connections between all three we gradually peel back the layers to a deeper understanding of who we are. The exercises in the second half of this book will focus on all three domains.

This is a simple model of the self. Figure 1.2 offers a more complex model which, whilst compatible with the first, opens up the domains and expands them. It incorporates Jung's work on the four functions of the mind; thinking, feeling, sensing and intuiting (Jung, 1978) and also an adaptation of Laing's concept of the real and false self, alluded to above. It also assimilates some of the aspects of self referred to in the discussion so far.

The model is divided into two parts. The outer public aspect of the self is what others see of us. The inner public aspect is what goes on in our heads and bodies. In one way, the outer experience is what other people are most familiar with. We communicate the inner experience through the outer. Our thoughts and feelings are all communicated through this outer presentation of self. Of what does it consist?

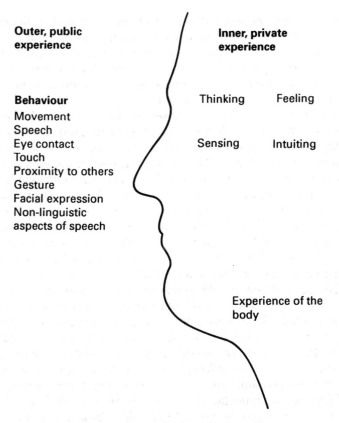

| Outer, public experience | | Inner, private experience |

Fig. 1.2 *A comprehensive model of the self*

The outer experience of the self

At the most obvious, behaviour consists of body movements; the turning of the head, the crossing of arms and legs, walking and running and so on. At a more subtle level the issue becomes more involved. We can note a whole variety of less obvious behaviours that convey something about the inner sense of self. First is speech. Clearly what we say, the words and phrase we use, are a potent means by which we convey thoughts and feelings to others. How we come to choose *these* particular words and phrases, however, depend on our past experiences, our education, our social position, our attitudes, values and beliefs and on the company that we are in when we use those words. Running alongside speech are the non-linguistic aspects of speech: timing, pacing, volume, minimal prompts ('mm's' and 'yes's'), the use of silence and so on. The use of such non-linguistic aspects of speech can be a powerful way of conveying our inner selves to others. As we noted above, we are always communicating—even when we think we are not!

When we talk to others we invariably look at them. As Heron (1970) notes there can be a wide variety in the intensity, amount and quality of eye contact. When we are embarrassed or upset, for example, we make less eye contact. When we are emotionally close to another person, our eye contact is often sustained. We can learn to become conscious of our use of what must be the most powerful aspect of communication and to monitor the amount and quality of our eye contact. We should also remain aware of the *cultural* differences that are involved here. People from cultures very different to our own use eye contact in other ways. It is important that we do not interpret such different use of eye contact inappropriately.

Touch in relation to others is another important aspect of our outer experience. Typically, in this culture, we touch more those people to whom we are close; members of the family, lovers and very close friends. Nursing involves a high degree of this personal aspect of human interaction and it is important that, as with eye contact, we learn to monitor and consciously use the facility of touch. It is worth noting, too, that some people are 'high touchers' and others 'low touchers'. Some people like being touched and like touching others; other people are repelled by it. Also, all touching should be unambiguous; clearly touch has sexual connotations for some people.

When we communicate verbally with others, we tend to stand or sit close to them. How near we stand or sit in relation to others is determined by a number of factors—the level of intimacy we have with them, our relationship with them and whether or not we are dominant or submissive in that relationship (Brown, 1965). In the nursing profession, nurses tend to be in a dominant position *vis a vis* their patients and will tend to stand closer to their patients than would be the case in ordinary day-to-day relationships. It is useful to imagine that we are surrounded by an invisible bubble, the threshold of which can only be crossed by certain other people. If people accidentally break through the bubble and touch us, they tend to withdraw quickly to avoid embarrassment to both parties. The issue of proximity to others needs close consideration. We need to become aware of how close or distant we like to be in relation to others. We need also to note other people's preferences and to be sensitive towards them. One useful way of judging this distance between you and the other person is to allow the other person to set that distance. In other words, you invite the other person to draw up a chair or you allow them to determine where *they* will stand in relation to you and not *vice versa*. Once again, as we become more self-aware, so we gain more insight into the needs and wants of others.

One of the clearest indicators of our inner experience is facial expression. Frowns and smiles do much to convey the feelings that are being experienced inside. It is important that facial expression and speech are congruent or matched. We have all experienced the person who *says* that they are cheerful or upset but whose facial expression suggests otherwise. Bandler and Grinder (1975) note that for the purposes of clear communication, three aspects of our outer behaviour must match; general body position, content of speech and facial expression. If two or more of these is mismatched then our communication will be confused and confusing. Thus, if we *say* that we are cheerful but shrug our shoulders and have an unhappy expression, the message will be unclear. We can do a lot to improve our communication on this level. It is insufficient just to *say* what we mean. We must be *seen* to mean it as well.

Two issues that become clear from this brief analysis of the outer aspects of self. We can become aware of our use of speech, eye contact, touch, proximity to others, gesture, facial expression and non-linguistic aspects of speech as a means of deepening our understanding of ourselves. Also, by becoming conscious of how we use those verbal and non-verbal behaviours we can use them more skilfully to enhance our contact with others. We can increase our interpersonal skills by intentionally using ourselves as instruments. Heron uses the expression 'conscious use of self' (Heron, 1973) to convey this concept. This is not to say that we need to become robotic and artificial but to note that in caring for others we can use more precisely our 'selves' as instruments of communication.

The Inner Experience

The inner, private experience in this model may be divided into four aspects of mental functioning—thinking, feeling, sensing and intuiting—and the experience of the body. Clearly, the division of these aspects into two groups is artificial as both mental and physical events are interrelated. As Searle (1983) points out, a mental event is also a physical event. To think that it is not is to perpetuate the old philosophical problem of mind/body dualism. This is sometimes know as Cartesian dualism after the philosopher Réne Descartes, who believed that mental and physical events could be considered separately. Today, the tendency is towards healing this split and interest continues to develop in concepts of holistic nursing and holistic medicine, both of which treat the mind and body together. As we have already noted, any concept of the self must take into account the mind and the body as a totality.

The thinking dimension

In this model, thinking refers to all the aspects, logical and otherwise, of our mental processes. One moments reflection on thinking will reveal that it is not a linear process. We do not think in sentences or even in a series of phrases. The process is much more haphazard than that. The technique known as 'free-association' as used in psychoanalysis demonstrates the apparently random nature of some of our thinking. Free association demands individuals to verbalize whatever comes into their mind, without any attempt at censoring or of stopping the flow. Try to attempt to do this. The process is always difficult and sometimes impossible. The reasons for this are outlined in the psychoanalytical literature and such a theory can offer insights into the genesis and nature of thought processes. Clearly, not everybody wants or can afford psychoanalysis but its ideas can be useful in attempting to understand thinking.

Arguably, the domain of thinking is more dominant in certain individuals. Certainly, thinking is highly rated in our culture and the education system sometimes seems to concern itself *only* with this mode. The domains of feeling, sensing and intuiting are usually less well catered for. In nursing, however, we are concerned with all sorts of feelings, from pain to anxiety, from depression to elation. Understanding these requires the use of dimensions other than thinking. On the other hand, it is obviously important that we all develop the thinking aspect. If we are to progress as a research-based-profession and if we are to be able to demonstrate critical awareness, we must be able to think clearly. We must also be able to appreciate when feeling gets in the way of thinking, as well as *vice versa*.

The feeling dimension

Feeling in this model refers to the emotional aspect of the person; love, sadness, joy, happiness etc. Heron (1977) argues that there are four dominant aspects of emotion that are frequently denied and repressed in our culture; anger, grief, fear and embarrassment. He argues that anger can be expressed through loud sound and shouting, grief through tears, fear through trembling and embarrassment through laughter. He argues further that such expression of emotion (or catharsis) is a healthy process. Heron claims that we live in a non-cathartic culture and the general tendency is to encourage people to control rather than to express emotion. As a result, we all carry round with us a pool of unexpressed emotion which distorts our thinking and stops us functioning fully. If we can learn to express some of this bottled up emotion (methods of doing this will be discussed later) then we can become more open to experience, less fearful and anxious and we can exercise more self-determination and autonomy. Part of becoming self-aware entails discovering and exploring the emotional dimension.

Nurses must deal with other people's emotions and there is a positive link between the way in which we handle our own emotions and the way in which we handle those of others. If we understand and can appropriately express our own anger, fear, grief and embarrassment, we will be better able to handle them in other people. In caring for others, we must get to know ourselves better.

Certainly other people's emotions affect us and stir up our own, unexpressed emotions. Try this simple experiment. Next time a programme on television moves you near to tears, turn off the set and allow yourself to cry. As you do so, reflect on what it is you are crying about. It is highly likely that the issue causing the tears is a personal one, not directly related to the television programme. Most people carry around with them this unexpressed emotion, just beneath the surface. Nurses who work in particularly emotionally charged environments—children's wards, intensive therapy units, psychiatric units and so forth—may want to consider self-help methods for exploring their own hidden emotions. Co-counselling, discussed in the next chapter is one such method and others are discussed by Bond (1986) and Bond and Kilty (1982). Alternatively, consider going to the cinema as a means of emotional release ... what do most people go to the cinema for? To cry, to allow themselves to get frightened or to laugh. The cinema and to a lesser extent, the theatre, concerts and sporting events offer 'natural' release valves for people's pent up emotion.

The sensing dimension

The sensing dimension in the model refers to inputs through the five special senses; touch, taste, smell, hearing, sight and also to proprioceptive and kinaesthetic sense. Proprioception refers to our ability to know the position of our bodies and thus to know where we are in space. We do not, for instance, need to *think* about our body position most of the time. We are fed that information by bundles of nerve fibres know as proprioceptors. Kinaesthetic sense refers to our sense of body movement. Again, this is not a sense that we normally have to think about.

We can make ourselves aware of any of the senses. Another simple experiment will demonstrate this. Stop reading for a moment and pay attention to everything that you can hear. Take in all the sounds around you, the more subtle as well as the more obvious. In doing so, notice how much of this one particular sense is normally passed over and how many sounds are usually filtered out of consciousness. At times it is vital that our senses are selective and that extraneous sounds, images, smells and so on are banished from awareness. On the other hand, the filtering mechanism often becomes too efficient and we filter out or fail to notice many sounds and sights that are around us all the time. We live half asleep.

In developing an awareness of our senses, we can begin to notice the world again. Just as importantly, we can begin to notice *each other* again. In developing our sense of sight, for instance, we can begin to notice subtle changes in other people's expressions, body postures and other aspects of non-verbal communication. Without that awareness we may miss a considerable amount of essential interpersonal information. In nursing, the value of such awareness is clear. Nurses need to be observant. What is not always so clear is *how* nurses are supposed to become observant. Like the development of any other skill, training to notice takes time and practice. The redeeming feature is that it is a skill which *individuals* can develop for themself. In a way, it is simply a matter of *remembering* to notice. Eventually, such awareness or 'staying awake' becomes part of the person.

The intuitive dimension

The intuitive dimension is perhaps the most undervalued. Intuition refers to knowledge and insight that arrives independently of the senses. In other words we just 'know'. Ornstein (1975) who studies the literature on the differences between the two sides of the brain identified intuition with the right side. He argued that the two sides have qualitatively different functions. The left side is concerned with cognitive processes and with rationality. According to Ornstein the right is more to do with holism, creativity and intuition. If he is right, the implication is that if the intuitive aspect is developed further (along with creativity) then both sides of the brain will function optimally. Ornstein argues that the present Western culture is dominated by the left brain approach to education and development. He calls for an educational system that honours creativity and intuition *alongside* the development of rationality.

Perhaps we neglect intuition through fear of it or concern that it may not be trusted. On the other hand, it is likely that we all have 'hunches' that when followed turn out to be 'right'. Many aspects of nursing require the nurse to be intuitive. Sometimes, in order to empathize with another person we have to guess at what they are feeling. Sometimes we seem to 'know' what they are feeling. Certainly, group work and counselling depend to a fair degree on this intuitive ability. Carl Rogers, founder of client-centred counselling noted that when he had a hunch about something that was happening in a counselling session, it invariably helped if he verbalized that intuition (Rogers, 1967). Using intuition consciously and openly takes courage and sometimes it is wrong. On the other hand, used along with more traditional forms of thinking, it can enhance the nurse/patient relationship in a way that logic on its own, never can.

The experience of the body

The third aspect of the model of self-awareness is the experience of the body. If the mind and body are directly interrelated, in fact inseparable, then any mental activity will affect the body and *vice versa*. It is notable, however, that much of the literature in nursing and medicine divides the person up into separate psychological and physiological entities. Indeed the two spheres are treated, typically, by different practitioners; general nurses care for physical ailments and psychiatric nurses for psychological problems. All this may change with the implementation of the guidelines in Project 2000 which may help to marry the two aspects of self back together via nurses studying the whole person.

It is easy to talk as though the mind and body *were* separate. Indeed we do not have a mind/body, we *are* our mind/body. Everything that we refer to as being part of our mind and body is part of our selves. Expressions such as 'I'm not happy with my body ...' or 'I've got that sort of mind ...' indicate how easy it is for us to dissociate ourselves from either the body or the mind.

Coming to notice body feelings takes time and patience. Of course, appreciation of inner bodily experiences are limited to some degree by the supply of sensory nerve endings to certain aspects of the body. Some parts are better served than others. On the other hand it is easy to lose touch with those bodily sensations of which we *may* become aware. Before you read any further, just take a moment to notice what is going on inside your body. What do you notice? Are there areas of muscle tension? Are the muscles of your stomach pulled in tightly? Can you become aware of your breathing? Are you breathing deeply into your stomach or is your breathing light and shallow? What happens when you make small changes to your body? What happens when you relax sets of muscles or change your breathing?

All of the information that can be gleaned from the body can enable us to appreciate something about our psychological status. Tension in sets of muscles, for example, may be the first we know of the fact that we are anxious or tense. Learning to 'listen' to the body in this way can help us to assess more accurately our true feelings about ourselves and others. Wilhelm Reich (1949), a psychoanalyst who was particularly interested in the mind/body relationship, advanced the notion of 'character armour'. Reich maintained that our emotional feelings could become trapped within sets of muscles and consequently affected posture and movement. He suggested that direct manipulation of those sets of muscles could release the emotion trapped within them with characteristic emotional release of catharsis. Such work on the body has become known as Reichian bodywork (Totton and Edmonston, 1988) and can be a powerful and effective means of developing self-awareness through direct body contact.

Similar but different methods of this sort which involve direct physical contact include Rolfing (Rolf, 1973), bioenergetics (Lowen, 1967) and Feldenkrais (Feldenkrais, 1972), three bodywork methods that have developed out of Reich's original formulation. Less dramatic but valid methods of body/mind exploration include; massage, yoga, the martial arts, certain types of meditation, the Alexander technique (Alexander, 1969), dance and certain types of sport. Examples of meditatitive techniques are included in the second half of this book.

All these methods can enhance awareness of self through attention to changes in the body and thus create insight into psychological states. They can also aid the development of awareness of body image. Observations of people in everyday life will reveal how frequently people walk around with lop-sided shoulders, a stooping gait or even with either side of their face showing different expressions. Often, too, they seem to be totally unaware of these things. Bodywork methods can enable the individual to develop greater physical symmetry and balance, better posture, improved breathing and a healthier physical status, generally. All aspects of nursing call for psychological and physical stamina and are taxing on the mind/body. These methods in combination with more traditional approaches to self-awareness can lead to a powerful and healthy approach to self-care. Perhaps burnout, so frequently a problem of occupations that depend upon a high degree of human contact, can be prevented effectively through this mix of attention to the body and mind.

Self-awareness

A model of the self has been outlined which takes account of the inner and outer aspects of the concept and which has attempted to marry the mind and body. The question now arises; what is self-awareness?

A first point that needs to be made is that what is *not* being discussed is 'self-consciousness', in the everyday sense of the word. To be self-conscious is to be embarrassed by ourselves, to be painfully aware of our being observed by others. Sartre (1956) describes this well when he suggests that under the scrutinizing gaze of the other person, we are turned into an object, a 'thing'. It is our response to being treated in this way that causes us to become self-conscious. For very self-conscious persons, this sense of being treated as an object is exaggerated by the persons themself. In being too acutely aware of other people's attention, she imagines herself to be more acutely scrutinized than is actually the case. It is rather like having someone watch us undertaking a skill such as giving an injection. We tend to (a) become deskilled by their watching us and (b) imagine that they are being highly critical. Self-consciousness is a bit like this. It tends to make you awkward and tends to make you feel criticized. This is true, for example of the adolescent who imagines (usually falsely) that they are being looked at with highly critical eyes. Their own sense of insecurity is projected onto the world and they imagine that others view them as harshly and as critically as they view themselves.

Clearly, such self-consciousness is more of a hindrance than a help when it comes to relating to others, as any acutely shy person knows. Yet such self-consciousness is far removed from self-awareness and may indicate a false or exaggerated self-concept.

Self-awareness refers to the gradual and continuous process of noticing and exploring aspects of the self, whether behavioural, psychological or physical, with the intention of developing personal and interpersonal understanding. Such awareness is probably best not developed for its own sake; it is intimately bound up with our relationships with others. To become more aware of and to have a deeper understanding of ourselves is to have a sharper and clearer picture of what is happening to others. In this sense, it is a process of discrimination. The more we can discriminate ourselves from others, the more we can understand our similarities. If we are unaware and blind to our own selves then we are likely to remain blind to others. A rather crude illustration may help to drive this point home. If I buy a red sweater, I immediately notice how many other people are wearing red sweaters—a fact of which I was not aware before the purchase. In noticing that fact about others I can also notice other things about them. And so, if I let it, the process escalates. I can notice more subtle differences between persons but also their similarities. The point is that the process begins with me. I must first examine myself.

Such a process of examination requires patience and honesty. It is easy to fall into the trap of *interpreting* thoughts, feelings and behaviour, rather than (initially at least) merely noticing them. That interpretation logically comes after we have gathered the data, *after* we have clearly described to ourselves our present status. This stage of self-awareness training may be likened to the assessment stage of the nursing process. Information about the self is gathered in order to develop a clearer picture, before any attempt is made to problem solve, decide upon changes, or identify reasons for the way we are.

This approach may be described as a phenomenological one (Spinelli 1989). Phenomenology is a branch of philosophy that is concerned with attempting to *describe* things as they appear to be without recourse to making value-judgements about them. Thus, in the human context, a phenomenological approach to self-awareness training would concern itself purely with *describing* aspects of the self as they surface and become known. Such an approach demands that we suspend judgement on ourselves. Instead of telling ourselves that 'this bit of me is O.K., this bit is bad and needs to be changed', we merely note that it *is as it is*. Once we have more data at our disposal, the answer to the question 'why?' may become self-evident. To jump to hasty conclusions may be either a) to be harshly critical of ourselves or b) to wreck the project altogether because we are disenchanted. Certainly, the road to self-awareness is not an easy one to tread, but the phenomenological approach can make it bearable. After all, if we don't accept ourselves, who will? If we don't accept ourselves, will we accept other people?

This method of description rather than interpretation is of great value in group settings and in counselling. When experiential learning is discussed in the next chapter, the notion of the phenomenological role of the facilitator is described. In this role, the facilitator of the group does not attempt to offer interpretations of what is happening in the group but limits descriptions to events and behaviours and encourages other group members to do the same. In the context of counselling, the phenomenological approach also pays dividends. If we can stand back and avoid interpreting what it is we think our clients are saying, we give them the chance to make their own interpretations. This attitude towards counselling is known as the client-centred approach (Rogers, 1967; Burnard, 1989). It is argued that the only people who *can* make a valid interpretation of their behaviour is the person, themself.

Developing self-awareness

There are various ways of developing self-awareness. Some involve introspection and some entail involvement with and feedback from other people. Any course leading towards self-awareness must contain both facets; the inner search and the observations of others.

Introspection by itself can lead to a one-sided, totally subjective view of the self. It is difficult, if not impossible, for the person working on her own to transcend herself and take the larger view. In order to balance that subjective view, we need the view of others.

Before examining some of the methods of introspection and group work, it is useful to note one simple method of enhancing self-awareness: the process of noticing what we are doing, the process of self-monitoring. All that is involved here is that you stay conscious of what you are doing, as you do it. In other words, you 'stay awake' and develop the skill of keeping your attention focused on your actions, both verbal and non-verbal. Such a process, whilst easy in theory can, in practice be quite difficult. It is easy to become distracted by inner thoughts and preoccupations so that our actions become automatic and unnoticed, even robotic. At this point it may be useful to examine three zones of attention on which we can focus.

Figure 1.3 shows these three, hypothetical zones. Zone 1 is the zone of having our attention focused 'out', on to our behaviour or on to the world outside ourselves. This is the zone being described above. To stay awake is to have attention focused outwards. There are some simple devices, borrowed from meditation that can encourage, enhance or develop our ability to keep our attention in that zone. Here is a straightforward one. Stop reading for a moment and allow your eyes to focus on an object in the room that you are in: it may be a piece of furniture, a picture or anything else that is to hand. Focus your attention on that object and notice every detail of it; its shape, its texture, its colour and so on. Continue to do this for about 30 seconds. Then discontinue your close observation. Notice how, whilst doing the exercise, your attention has been drawn away from your own thoughts and feelings to enable you to focus fully on the object.

The practice of this simple exercise can help in getting and keeping attention *out*. If we do not focus out, we do not fully notice ourselves and others. Instead, we give half of our attention to ourselves or others and are not really 'present' for either. When we have our attention out, we can give ourselves more fully to what we are doing, to give our attention more fully to the person we are with.

Zones 2 and 3 in Fig. 1.3 are the zones of introspection. Inward focusing of attention (or *attention in*) can be useful as a means of exploring thoughts, feelings or bodily sensations. Access to Zone 2 is very straightforward. Stop reading and close your eyes. Allow your attention to range freely over what is going on in your mind. Notice

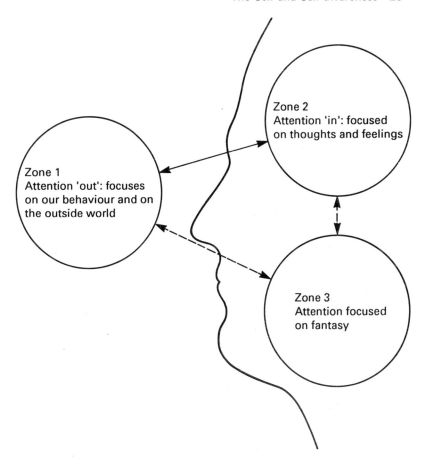

Fig. 1.3 *Zones of awareness*

the things that you are thinking; notice how you are feeling and pay attention to any body sensations that you have. What parts of your body are you aware of? What parts can you not sense at all? Is there anything you can do in order to become aware of those parts of your body? After one or two minutes, open your eyes and switch your focus back to the outside world. Notice whether such a switch is easy or difficult. The ability to shuttle between Zones 1 and 2 can be developed through practice.

Zone 3 involves fantasy. Fantasy refers to all our thoughts and feelings that involves imagining or day-dreaming; anything that is not *fact*. Notice how we often have fantasies about both ourselves and others that are in no way related to fact. We *imagine* for instance what other people think of us. We *imagine* what sorts of people other people are. We *guess* at what they are thinking about or what they think of us. In each case we are dealing, not with how things *are* but *how we imagine them to be*. Often these imaginings or fantasies are based on the flimsiest of evidence. Often they are pure fantasy—they have no grounding in fact at all! Differentiating between Zones 2 and 3 is particularly fruitful. Such differentation allows us to distinguish between what we know and what we *think* we know. If we acknowledge when we are moving from the zones of logical, clear thinking (Zone 2) to the zone of fantasy (Zone 3), we develop a clearer picture of what goes on inside our heads. This is not to denigrate the zone of fantasy, for it can be a rich source of creativity and inspiration. It is just to note that fantasy is always just that; it can never be reality.

Awareness of our focus of attention and its shift between the three zones has implications for all aspects of nursing. The nurse who is able to keep her attention focused out for longer periods is likely to become more observant and more accurate in those observations. The nurse who can differentiate between the zones of thinking and the zones of fantasy is less likely to jump to conclusions about her observations or to make value judgements based on prejudice rather than on fact. She is also likely to be more effective as a critical thinker and more able to assess and evaluate new ideas and new theories.

The study of the three zones can never be exhaustive. To explore Zone 1 is also to explore the outer aspect of self; our behaviour, speech and so on. It is also to explore the environment in which we live and move. It is to come to know more about the world around us and the people who share it with us.

To explore Zone 2 is also a job for life. There would seem to be no end to how much we can study our thought processes, feeling states and bodily sensations. Likewise, examining our fantasy life can give us insights into the sorts of people we are, how we picture ourselves, others and the world around us.

All such explorations can be carried out either in isolation, with another person or in groups. To explore the self in the company of another person can be a rewarding and economical method. Economical in that the time available can be equally divided between the two people. Co-counselling offers a useful format for such exploration and this is explained in the next chapter.

Other methods of self-awareness training include the use of role-

Possible aspects of self-awareness	Practical methods of developing aspects of self-awareness
1. Thoughts, including: (a) stream of consciousness (b) ideas (c) fantasy (d) delusions/false beliefs (e) recurrent thought patterns, etc.	1. Discussion/conversation/group work 2. Introspection 3. Meditation 4. Brainstorming exercises 5. Co-counselling 6. Writing 7. Use of problem-solving strategies, etc.
2. Feelings, including: (a) anger (b) fear (c) grief (d) embarrassment (e) joy, happiness, etc.	1. Discussion/conversation/ group work 2. Introspection 3. Meditation 4. Gestalt exercises 5. Co-counselling 6. Counselling/therapy 7. Psychodrama 8. Role-play 9. Cathartic exercises 10. Encounter/sensitivity training, etc.
3. Spirituality, including: (a) clarification of belief systems (b) life philosophy (c) awareness of choice of expression, of spiritual needs, etc.	1. Discussion/conversation/ group work 2. Meditation 3. Prayer 4. Aesthetic experience (e.g. art, music, etc.) 5. Reading 6. Life-planning, etc.
4. Sensation, including (a) taste (b) touch (c) smell (d) hearing (e) sight (f) kinaesthetic (g) proprioceptive, etc.	1. Focussing attention on one or more sensation(s) 2. Group exercises 3. Use of sensory stimulation/ deprivation 4. Gestalt exercises, etc.
5. Sexuality, including: (a) orientation (heterosexual, homosexual, bisexual) (b) expression, etc.	1. Discussion/conversation/group work 2. Counselling/co-counselling 3. Values, clarification exercises, etc.

Possible aspects of self-awareness	Practical methods of developing aspects of self-awareness
6. Physical status, including: (a) the body systems (b) status in terms of health/illness (c) the link between emotional and physical status, etc.	1. Self examination 2. Medical examination 3. Autogenic training 4. Exercise 5. Yoga, Tai Chi, etc. 6. Meditation 7. Massage 8. Alexander technique 9. Reichian bodywork, etc.
7. Appearance, including (a) dress (b) personal style (c) height, weight, etc.	1. Discussion/conversation/group work 2. Self and peer assessment 3. Self-monitoring 4. Video, etc.
8. Knowledge, including: (a) subjective, 'personal' knowledge (b) objective 'public' knowledge (c) gaps in knowledge, etc.	1. Discussion/conversation/group work 2. Examination/testing/quizzing 3. Brainstorming 4. Self- and peer-assessment 5. Reading/studying 6. Use of journals/diaries, etc.
9. Practical, interactive and technical skills, including: (a) listening skills (b) counselling skills (c) group skills (d) range of practical skills, etc.	1. Discussion/conversation/group work 2. Role play 3. Video 4. Social skills training exercises 5. Counselling skills training exercises, etc.
10. Needs and wants, including: (a) financial/material (b) physical (c) love and belonging (d) achievement (e) knowledge (f) aesthetic (g) spiritual (h) self-actualisation, etc.	1. Discussion/conversation group work 2. Values clarification exercises 3. Life style evaluation 4. Brainstorming and use of problem-solving cycle, etc.
11. Dreams	1. Maintenance of dream journal 2. Dream, analysis (e.g. gestalt, Jungian, etc.) etc.

Possible aspects of self-awareness	Practical methods of developing aspects of self-awareness
12. Verbal activity, including: (a) use of particular words or phrases (b) active and latent vocabulary (c) accent, pronunciation (d) use of silence, etc.	1. See below, under 13.
13. Non-verbal activity, including: (a) facial expression (b) eye contact (gaze) (c) gestures (d) proximity to others (e) use of touch (f) body position/posture, etc.	1. Discussion/conversation/group work 2. Video 3. Role play/psychodrama 4. Self- and peer-assessment 5. Use of mirrors 6. 'Conscious use of self', etc.
14. Self, in relation to others, including: (a) feeling for others (b) ability to give attention (c) confidence/lack of confidence with others, etc.	1. Discussion/conversation/group work 2. Assertion training exercises 3. Counselling training exercises 4. Social skills training 5. Co-counselling, etc.
15. Values, including (a) values system (b) moral code (c) open/closed mindedness (d) areas of prejudice, etc.	1. Discussion/conversation group work 2. Values clarification exercises 3. Use of rating scales, etc.
16. Unknown/undiscovered aspects, including: (a) subpersonalities (b) transpersonal aspects (c) unconscious aspects, etc.	1. Self-disclosure 2. Co-counselling 3. Transactional analysis 4. Self-analysis/psychoanalysis, etc.

Fig. 1.4 *Methods of developing self-awareness*

play, social skills training, meditation and assertiveness skills training. These methods are well documented in the literature (see for example, Kagan, 1985; Hargie, et al., 1987; Bond 1986; Burnard 1989) and courses in these forms of training are frequently organized by women's groups, growth centres and extra-mural departments of colleges and universities.

In nurse education and training, the use of video can enhance self-awareness by allowing students to view themselves as if from another person's point of view. Such training, however, should always be voluntary. Some people find the use of video tapping a gross invasion of personal territory and the method should be used with discretion.

As we have noted, work on the body via Reichian body work, yoga, tai chi, the martial arts and sport all have their place in self-awareness development both for their effects on the body but also for their limit-testing capacity. A quieter, more reflective approach is the use of journals or diaries and these can be used to monitor self-awareness development alongside educational development.

Probably the ideal is a combination of a variety of approaches; introspection, with a group, active and passive. In this way, the self is studied in all its aspects and in a variety of contexts, As we have noted, the 'self' is not a static once-and-for-all thing but an entity that is constantly changing depending amongst other things, on the people we are with. The eclectic approach is also healthier in that it encourages the combination of sport and exercise alongside meditation and more reflective practices. It also allows for normal social relationships to develop alongside periods of solidarity. No one ever became self-aware by shutting themselves away from the rest of the world. Also, it is important that self-awareness development has a practical end—the enhancement of interpersonal relationships and skills.

Figure 1.4. maps our the wide variety of aspects of self-awareness and some of the methods that can be used in the development of such awareness. It is not exhaustive of all possible methods, nor is it hierarchical in nature; no one aspect of self-awareness is deemed to be more or less important than any other.

Self-awareness and the nurse

Having explored the concept of self and examined some methods of self-awareness development, the question remains: why develop self-awareness anyway?

In the first instance, to discover more about ourselves is to differentiate ourselves from others. If we cannot differentiate between *our own* thoughts and feelings and those of others, we stand to blur our ego boundaries, our sense of ourself as an independent, autonomous being. Conversely, if we constantly blur the distinction between 'you and me' we risk not recognising the other person's independence and autonomy. When ego boundaries are blurred, we loose the sense of whose problem is whose. With self-awareness we can learn to distinguish between our problems and those of others and *vice versa*. This is particularly important in sensitive areas such as psychiatry and care of the dying person. Real involvement and care in these fields also involves (almost paradoxically) the ability to detach ourselves a little in order to get things into perspective. If we cannot engage in this distancing we risk being drawn into other people's problems to such a degree that we can no longer help them. *Their* problems, have become *ours*.

To become self-aware is also to learn conscious use of the self. We become agents; we are able to choose to act rather than feeling acted upon. We learn to select therapeutic interventions from a range of options so that the patient or client benefits more completely. If we are blind to ourselves we are also blind to our choices. We are blind then, to caring and therapeutic choices that we could make on behalf of our patients.

Once we can combine two aspects—differentiation from others and an increase awareness of the range of therapeutic choices available to use—we can be more sensitive to the needs and wants of others. We can even choose to *forget ourselves* in order to give ourselves more completely to others. No longer do we run the risk of getting sucked into other people's problems, nor do we confuse *our* thoughts and feelings with those of our patients. We can offer therapeutic distance with therapeutic choice.

Interpersonal interventions such as counselling and group facilitation require that we exercise some self-awareness. All that has been discussed in the above paragraphs is particularly true when we are trying to help people in these particular sorts of therapeutic situations. In part two of this book, both counselling skills and group facilitation skills are explored. It is a vital prerequisite that alongside the development of such skills, the person taking part in the activities in this section will also continue to develop self-awareness. Skills development without self awareness tends to encourage the development of a stilted and unnatural presentation of self. Without self-awareness, the person appears merely to have a set of skills 'tacked on'; those skills are used neither sensitively nor awarely but in a robotic and automatic way.

Problems in self-awareness development

It is worth repeating the point made at various stages throughout this chapter; that the aim of self-awareness development is to enable us to increase our interpersonal skills. The path to such awareness is, however, fraught with problems. First is the problem of egocentricity. It is possible to become caught up in the idea of understanding the self to the degree that it becomes an end in itself. This tends to lead to the person becoming self-indulgent and self-centred. Clearly such positions are not compatible with altruism or concern for others. Second, it is possible for those who develop self-awareness to believe that they have discovered insights that set them apart or even make them better than other people. A sign of such development is sometimes the loss of a sense of humour. Life becomes very earnest. True self-awareness, however, tends to lead to a lightness of touch and a sense of humility at the sheer vastness of the task in hand. To continue with that task, it is important that the person maintains (and exercises) a sense of humour in order to keep sight of the 'larger canvas'. Certainly the best run self-awareness groups are those that offer a 'light' atmosphere. If the atmosphere becomes too heavy and earnest, it is likely to put everyone off. It is certainly not conducive to easy and frank self-disclosure.

Linked to this, is the problem of the self-awareness group facilitator becoming something of a 'guru' figure. As people find things out about themselves, they sometimes tend to imagine that the group facilitators have special qualities that enable them to allow this to happen. As a result, those people tend to set the facilitator up as some sort of hero. Sometimes, too, the facilitator believes in this image and ends up acting out the role of guru. Again, caution and humility are keywords. Both group members and facilitator should remember that the facilitator is human, like everyone else. In my experience (and for whatever reason) it is nearly always men who either set themselves up in the guru role or are set up in it by their groups.

Finally comes the issue of voluntariness. Self-awareness cannot be forced upon people. Facilitators of self-awareness groups would do well to exercise what Heron (1977b) calls the voluntary principle. This is a principle invoked at the beginning of any self-awareness training course and repeated at intervals throughout such a course that no one at any time will have pressure exerted on them to take part and that everyone takes part in any exercise of their own free will. If self-awareness is about developing autonomy and the exercise of choice, it is important that such autonomy and choice begins with deciding whether or not a given exercise suits them at this time. Accepting and respecting other people's frailties, their reserve and their choice not to disclose aspects of themselves until they are ready, are all part of the process of facilitation. Such understanding on the part of the facilitator will do much to increase the confidence of group members and to create an atmosphere conducive to self-understanding.

2

Experiential Learning

> I can give you nothing that has not already its being
> within yourself. I can thrown open to you no
> picture-gallery but your own soul ... I help you to
> make your own world visible. That is all.
> (Hermann Hesse)

Experiential learning has become an important tool for the development of nursing skills (Kagan, Evans and Kay 1986; Tomlinson 1985; Miles 1987). This chapter explores the concept of experiential learning. The aim of this chapter is to explore the concept as it applies to nurse education and particularly as it applies to the development of interpersonal skills. It should be noted, at the outset, that the concept has been used in a wide variety of ways in the literature. Examples of the concepts which various writers have used in the context of experiential learning include, amongst others:

- learning by doing the job
- learning from life experience
- allowing people credits for their life experience in place of formal qualifications when applying for places at university
- adult education
- humanistic education
- education of feelings as well as thoughts
- progressive and radical educational methods
- education to increase political awareness
- non-formal education
- 'alternative' education
- the 'romantic' as opposed to the 'classical' curriculum.

The one thing that all of these various ways of approaching experiential learning have in common is the centrality of human experience as a valued source of learning. What follows is an attempt to explore ways in which we might learn from that experience. It is notable, too, that many of the writers who define experiential learning in so many different ways, tend to refer to the work of David Kolb (1984) whose experiential learning cycle will be examined in this chapter.

Learning By Experience

We all learn through experience, whether directly through taking action, through being involved in a situation or by observing others. In this sense, every situation is a potential learning situation. If we are not careful, the definition could become 'life equals experiential learning' and the definition would be so broad as to be of little meaning. It may be more helpful if we can pin it down a little more.

The first thing to note is that whilst every situation is a *potential* learning situation, we do not necessarily learn from everything we do or everything that we are involved in. Some sort of *cognitive* process is required; we need to notice what we do and we need to be aware of what is happening. Thus, the emphasis on self-awareness in the previous chapter. To learn more about ourselves (and then to learn about others), a basic requirement is that we *notice* ourselves. We need to be both *reflective* and able to notice what is happening around us and also *reflexive*, able to look inward and notice what we are thinking and feeling. Figure 2.1 offers a simple model of experiential learning which brings together these two notions of

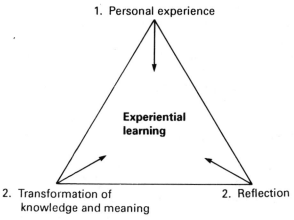

Fig. 2.1   *The concept of experiential learning*

experience followed by reflection and adds another ingredient: the transformation of knowledge.

First, the concept involves personal experience; the fact that something has happened to us, or our being actively involved in a situation. Such experience involves the whole of us; our thinking, feeling, behaving and bodily sense. The concept of personal experience can be loosely defined as our involvement in a situation.

The second element of experiential learning is the process of reflection. Often as something happens to us, we may have reason to ponder on it. We may not. Things may happen to us that we either do not notice or we quickly dismiss. Think for a moment of the times that you have driven (or been driven) from one place to another and then wondered how you had got from A to B. You did not realize what was happening because you did not *notice*; you were on 'automatic drive'. In experiential learning, the reflective process is vital. It is only through such reflection that we can ever achieve the third element: the transformation or knowledge and meaning.

Experiential learning can be characterized in at least two ways; a) as an attitude towards learning and b) as an approach to the question: what is knowledge? These two issues are now discussed.

An attitude towards learning

Many traditional methods of teaching and learning offer students large chunks of pre-packaged knowledge in indigestible chunks, upon which no reflection can take place. It is as if the object of learning was to be filled with knowledge, which can, at a later date be cashed out through examinations. Paulo Freire, the radical Marxist educator (Freire 1970; 1972) has referred to this as the 'banking' concept of knowledge. Knowledge is fed into the person, who reproduces it, later, in a relatively unchanged state. The main aim is to satisfy your educators that you have absorbed enough. Such an approach, apart from being fairly dull and unimaginative, presupposes a particular view of the nature of knowledge. From this traditional, 'banking' approach, aspects of knowledge are unchanging; 'facts are facts' and they exist independently of the one who does the 'knowing'. The process of education, then, is the initiation of the person into 'ways of knowing' (Peters, 1976). Educators are the 'ones who know' and students are the ones who don't. The educated person, presumably, is the one who has absorbed more knowledge than the rest.

An alternative approach is that which constantly questions knowledge. One of Marx's favourite aphorisms was 'doubt everything' (Singer, 1980) and this characterizes what Paulo Freire calls the 'problem-posing' approach to education (Freire, 1972). Rather than accepting everything that is passed on through traditional methods of teaching and learning, this approach emphasizes an approach to constantly questioning what is learnt through reference to *one's own* experience of the world. In other words, the 'received' view of the world is constantly called into question. Much of traditional nurse education has favoured the unquestioning acceptance of things as they are. The problem posing approach calls for challenge, doubt and an ability to question the established order to things. This ability to question the traditional and the accepted is demonstrated by two statements that Carl Rogers' makes (Rogers, 1967); 'I can trust my experience' and 'evaluation by others is not a guide for me'. Here, the accent is on finding out for ones' self, of testing out established theory through one's own experience.

How, then, can nurse educators encourage the development of critical ability? Drawing from and developing the work of Brookfield (1987), the following guidelines are offered:

a) Affirm critical thinkers' self worth. The critical thinker is an innovator, going out on a limb and trying to question the established order of things. They also challenge their own self-concept, for what we think and feel, as we have noted, constitutes our sense of self. We *are* our knowledge, feelings and actions. For these reasons, the critical thinker needs to be encouraged and made to feel that their ideas are appreciated and valued. In the exercises that follow, it is important that *unusual* ideas are also listened too.

b) Listen attentively to critical thinkers. Listening is an important aspect of nursing practice. We will see in the next chapter that it is one of the most important skills in counselling. It is also a vital prerequisite for helping to develop critical ability. When people express critical ideas, they are challenging the *status quo* and offering new views on a particular situation. The temptation is to react so as to bring the student back to the well-worn path. Facilitators who listen, however, develop the ability to follow a critical student's thought processes and enters their 'frame of reference' (Rogers, 1967). Such listening is always a challenge for what we may hear when listening to critical expression challenge, our own view of the world. This notion of an expanding frame of reference is at some variance with traditional views of education. Peters (1972) for example, argues that education is 'initiation into ways of knowing' and that the teacher's task is to lead the students into fields of study. In the version offered here, both students and teachers are co-travellers and develop their knowledge, feelings and skills alongside each other, challenging the other.

c) Be a critical teacher. A number of writers on education have discussed the notion of critical teaching. Shor (1980) defines critical teaching as assisting people to become aware of their taken-for-granted world. In the problem posing and critical approach to experiential learning, the facilitator acts as a catalyst, challenging the students to develop their new ideas and to question the world they find themselves in. Freire (1986) has suggested that the characteristics of such facilitators include competence, courage, risk-taking, humility and political clarity.

Setting out to engage in an experiential learning session of this sort is something of an act of faith. There is no way of knowing beforehand how such a session will end. Either students or facilitator, or both, may change their ideas as a result of the session. Facilitators who practice in this way 'live on the edge' and are prepared to take risks both with themself and with their students, in order to move thinking and feeling forward. The other important point here is that 'critical facilitation' does not involve the facilitator being critical of the students as might be the case in more traditional teaching. Indeed, the notion represents almost the opposite position. The facilitator is accepting the student but is prepared to question both her own and the student's ideas.

d) Model critical ability. If students are to learn to question and to criticize, it is important that facilitators demonstrate their own critical ability. This requires the facilitator to be open to new ideas, and to continue their own educational practice, and to be willing to learn from the students. Thus nurse education can become a reciprocal process, students and teachers switch roles throughout the educational process—a notion that Freire has also frequently referred to in his writings (Freire, 1970; 1972; 1985).

f) Learn to shut up! Most teachers of nurses talk too much. If facilitators are to encourage critical ability, students must have the chance to talk about what they think and feel. This cannot happen if the facilitator is talking. Further, silence has much to commend it. The notion that the facilitator must always 'fill in the gaps' during an educational encounter may be an erroneous one.

g) Be conversational. Much can be achieved if the facilitator adopts a fairly normal tone of voice and relates to students as equals and as interesting people with ideas of their own. Many interviews are spoiled by the artificial manner adopted by interviewers (Zweig, 1965). Many potential learning encounters are also spoiled by the teacher too zealously playing out a 'teacher role'. Much of the learning we do takes place outside of educational institutions (Illich, 1973) and this may because in everyday life, people talk to each other normally. A conversational exchange in the classroom can do much to enhance the free development of critical awareness in students. This notion of 'speaking normally' is an important one in experiential learning. In a field which has attracted a number of 'guru' figures, it is important that experiential learning facilitators take care not to mystify or otherwise worry their students.

Experiential Learning as the Development of Experiential Knowledge

Another approach to appreciating the notion of experiential learning comes through the notion of types of knowledge. Three types of knowledge that go to make up an individual may be described; propositional knowledge, practical knowledge and experiential knowledge (Heron, 1981). Whilst each of these types is different, each is interrelated with the other. Thus, whilst propositional knowledge is qualitatively different to for example, practical knowledge, it is possible and probably better to use propositional knowledge in the application of practical knowledge.

Propositional knowledge

Propositional knowledge is that which may be contained in theories or models. It may be described as 'textbook' knowledge and is synonymous with Ryle's (1949) concept of 'knowing that', which is a concept further developed in an educational context by Pring (1976). A person may build up a considerable bank of facts, theories or ideas about a subject, person or thing, without necessarily having any direct experience of that subject, person or thing. A person, may, for example develop a considerable propositional knowledge about, say, midwifery, without ever necessarily having been anywhere near a woman who is having a baby! Presumably it would be more useful to combine that knowledge with some practical experience, but this does not necessarily have to be the case. This then, is the domain of propositional knowledge. Obviously it is possible to have propositional knowledge about a great number of subject areas ranging from science to literature or from counselling to physiology. Any information contained in books must necessarily be of the propositional sort.

Practical knowledge

Practical knowledge is knowledge developed through the acquisition of skills. Thus changing a dressing or driving a motor bike demonstrates practical knowledge, although so does the use of counselling skills which involve the use of specific verbal and non-verbal behaviours and the intentional use of counselling interventions as described above. Practical knowledge is synonymous with Ryle's (1949) concept of 'knowing how' which was developed, in an educational context by Pring (1976). Usually more than mere 'knack', practical knowledge is the substance of a smooth performance of a practical or interpersonal skill. A considerable amount of a nurses's time is taken up with the demonstration of practical knowledge—often, but not always, of the interpersonal sort.

Most educational programmes in schools and colleges have concerned themselves primarily with both propositional and practical knowledge and particularly the former. Thus the 'propositional knowledge' aspect of a person is the aspect that is often held in highest regard. Practical knowledge, although respected, is usually seen as slightly less important than the propositional sort. In this way, the 'self' can become highly developed in one sense—the propositional knowledge aspect—at the expense of being skilled in a practical sense.

Experiential knowledge

Experiential knowledge is knowledge gained through direct encounter with a subject, person or thing. It is the subjective and affective nature of that encounter that contributes to this sort of knowledge. Experiential knowledge is knowledge through relationship. Such knowledge is synonymous with Roger's (1983) description of experiential learning and with Polanyi's concept of 'personal' knowledge and 'tacit' knowledge (Polanyi, 1958). If we reflect for a moment we may realize that most of the things that are really important to us belong in this domain. If we consider our personal relationships with other people, we discover that what we like or love about them cannot be reduced to a series of propositional statements and yet the feelings we have for them are vital and part of what is most important in our lives. Most encounters with others contain the possible seeds of experiential knowledge. It is only when we are so detached from other people that we treat them as objects that no experiential learning can occur.

Not that all experiential knowledge is tied exclusively to relationships with other people. For example, I had propositional knowledge about America before I went there. When I went there, all that propositional knowledge was changed considerably. What I had known was changed by my direct experience of the country. I had developed experiential knowledge of the place. Experiential knowledge is not of the same type or order as propositional or practical knowledge. It is, nevertheless, important knowledge, in that it affects everything else we think about or do.

Experiential knowledge is necessarily personal and idiosyncratic. Indeed, as Rogers (1983) points out, it may be difficult to convey to another person in words. Words tend to be loaded with personal (often experiential) meanings and thus to understand each other we need to understand the nature of the way in which the people with whom we converse use words. It is arguable, however, that such experiential knowledge is sometimes conveyed to others through gesture, eye contact, tone of voice, inflection and all the other non-verbal and paralinguistic aspects of communication (Argyle, 1975). Indeed, it may be experiential knowledge that is passed on when two people (for example nurses and their patient) become very involved with each other in a conversation, a learning encounter or counselling.

From the above discussion of three types of knowledge, it is possible to define experiential learning another way as, *any learning activity which enhances the development of experiential knowledge.* As with all interpersonal relationships, both within and without, of the health care professions, they involve an investment of the self, it seems reasonable to argue that any learning method that involves the self and that involve personal knowledge are likely to enhance personal effectiveness. We cannot, after all, learn interpersonal skills by rote, nor merely by mechanically learning a series of behaviour. We need to spend time reflecting on ourselves and on receiving feedback on our performance from other people.

Learning Through and Learning From Experience

Yet another way of understanding the concept of experiential learning is by the division of *learning through* experience and *learning from* experience. In learning through experience, a situation is set up that allows us to gain insight through participation. In learning *from* experience, we are required to look back at a past situation in our lives in order to glean new meanings from it and to compare it to our present situation. Both types of experiential situation may help us to think critically and carefully about ourselves, our nursing practice and about the *theories* that other people offer us.

Examples of situations that involve learning *through* experience and learning *from* experience are listed in Fig 2.2. Allied to these experiences are those activities that may be described as *experiential learning methods* (Fig 2.3). All of these encourage to a greater or lesser degree either reflection on past experience or fresh experience in the present.

The Characteristics of Experiential Learning

It is useful to identify the characteristics that consistently emerge from the theory and practice of experiential learning. These are as follows:

- There is an emphasis on action
- Students are encouraged to reflect on their experience
- A clarifying approach is adopted by the facilitator
- There is an accent on personal experience
- Human experience is valued as a source of learning.

These characteristics are now examined in order to make further sense of the concept of experiential learning. We have already noted the diversity of the definitions of experiential learning in the literature but these characteristics seem to permeate most approaches to the topic.

There is an emphasis on action

Most experiential learning methods involve the participants in some form of action. This is not to say that they are 'doing something' in a trivial sense but that they are learning through the processes of activity and movement. This can be viewed as the opposite of

Learning *THROUGH* experience	Learning *FROM* experience
1. Taking other people's and having one's own blood pressure taken	1. Reflection on childhood experiences
2. Lying in a hospital out-patients' department	2. Recall of first experiences at school
3. Lying in a hospital bed	3. Discussion of hospital experience as a patient
4. Being fed by a colleague	4. Recall of being interviewed by a doctor
5. Being dressed by a colleague	5. Reflection on relationships with parents.
6. Being lifted by colleagues	6. Recall of a specific happy incident from home life.
7. Being blindfolded and led by a colleague	7. Discussion of past job experiences
8. Visiting the GP	8. Reflection on the experience of bereavement
9. Undertaking certain experiential learning activities	9. Undertaking certain experiential learning activities

Fig 2.2 *Examples of situations for learning THROUGH and FROM experience*

traditional teaching/learning strategies which require the learner to be a passive recipient of received knowledge. Through activity we are engaged in learning through all of our senses, not merely in some sort of thinking process. In another sense too, experiential learning should *lead* to action. If our behaviour does not change as a result of our learning (particularly in the domain of interpersonal skills) then it is arguable that the learning has not been particularly valuable. Also, as we become more critically aware, we will tend to question more and thus want to change what we find in the clinical and community settings.

Group discussions
One-to-one exercises
Role Paly
Psychodrama
Co-Counselling activities
Simulation
Meditation
Relaxation exercises
Problem solving activities
Games
Guide fantasy
Encounter activities
Structured activities
Counselling exercises
Group facilitation exercises
Coaching
Clinical teaching

Fig 2.3   *Examples of experiential learning methods*

Students are encouraged to reflect on their experience

Most writers in the field acknowledge that experience alone is not sufficient to ensure that learning takes place. Importance is placed on the integration of new experience with old through the process of reflection (Kolb 1984, Kilty 1982; Freire 1972). In order to learn at all, we must be able to reflect on what we do and to undertake some sort of critical appraisal of what we find. The word 'critical' here is used to denote the process by which we ponder, sift, analyse and evaluate, it should not be taken as meaning only 'to judge negatively'.

Reflection can be a solitary, introspective act or it can be a group process whereby sense is made of an experience through group discussion. If reflection as a group activity is to be successful, the teacher is required to act as a group facilitator. The skills associated with group facilitation differ from those associated with the usual process of teaching in that the group facilitator takes a non-directive and non-authoritarian stance in relation to the students. In a reflective group, the teacher neither ascribes meanings to experience nor offers explanations but allows and encourages the students to do these things for themselves.

A clarifying approach is adopted by the tutor

In the experiential approach, the teacher does not 'teach' in the traditional sense, he or she does not dispense knowledge or force their meanings onto the student's experience (Gray, 1986). Instead, the teacher helps the students to make sense of their *own* experience. After an exercise in which students practice counselling skills, the teacher encourages quiet reflection on the exercise. Rather than offering explanations for what the students have undergone, the facilitator invites each student to comment on what happened and invites individuals and the group to 'make sense' of what happened. The teacher may help the students to verbalize their feelings and ideas but does not attempt to direct them. The teacher may, however, want to challenge them to consider *other* ways of construing what they have experienced. Thus, *challenging* is an approach to encourage the students to think in alternative and different ways (Brookfield, 1987). It is vital to critical development. This is not to suggest that the facilitator says 'But there is another way to see this ... here is another theory ...' Instead, the teacher merely asks something like 'Are there other ways of looking at this ...?' and waits for the students to bring forward other perspectives.

All this is not easy! Teachers, perhaps by nature, like telling students about their own particular experiences or theories. Probably most teachers talk too much. To stand back and allow personal discovery and personal theory development in this way is often to go against the traditional role of the teacher.

Through this process of clarification and critical development, nurses may develop an ability to trust their own judgement and to accept the validity of their own ideas, whilst respecting and appreciating other points of view. They do not strive towards *the* point of view. Nor do they have to defer to the better judgement or knowledge of the teacher but appreciate the value of their own thoughts and feelings about their experiences, both in the school or college and in clinical settings. In this sense, the nurse educator acts as a true 'facilitator of learning'. In the literature on experiential learning, the term 'facilitator' is often used in preference to the terms teacher, tutor and lecturer.

There is an accent on personal experience

Alfred North Whitehead discussed the problem of 'dead' knowledge and asserted that 'knowledge keeps no better than fish!' (Whitehead,

1932). Someone else has described formal teaching as the 'dragging a set of old bones from one graveyard to another' (Anon).

Experiential learning emphasizes the evolving, dynamic, nature of knowledge. Rather than viewing knowledge as fixed and immutable, it stresses the importance of the student understanding and creating a view of the world in that student's own terms. Knowledge, then, is not something that is 'tacked on' to the person; it becomes part of the person themselves. What we learn changes our world view and changes us. We are what we know. This is what is meant by the accent on personal experience.

As a nurse continues through education and training, what she learns becomes part of her. The nurse who becomes skilled at discussing problems with clients or patient changes as a result: the very personal experience of developing human skills helps the nurse towards an enhanced self-concept.

The Development of Experiential Learning Methods

Experiential learning methods have evolved from two main sources. One is from the theorizing of the American pragmatic philosopher, John Dewey. Dewey argues that all educational processes should be based on the life experiences of the students and that school experiences and life experiences should be directly linked in a planned programme. Dewey was the founder of the 'progressive' school of educational thought as opposed of the 'traditional' school which stressed the importance of academic disciples and the impartiality of knowledge. In stressing the importance of life experience as the foundation for the learning process, Dewey anticipated the work of Carl Rogers, Malcolm Knowles and other writers who democratized and personalized learning theory. His emphasis on practicality, the value of experience and the use of the student's own theorizing, made him a key figure in the history of experiential learning theory (Dewey 1966; 1958; 1971).

The second source from which many experiential learning methods are derived is the school of humanistic psychology. Humanistic psychology developed as a 'third force' in psychology in the 1950's and 1960's. The other two forces were behaviourism and psychoanalysis. Humanistic psychology opposed behaviourism on the grounds that it took a mechanistic view of the human being (although some have argued that the two approaches may be compatible [Woolfolk and Sass 1989]). Psychodynamic psychology was viewed as being overly deterministic (a deterministic theory is one that argues that present events are necessarily caused by previous events. Thus, for the psychoanalyst, we are a product of our past). Humanistic psychology opposed this determinism, arguing the idea that people were able to exercise free will and to some degree *choose* who they were. In other words, the person was an 'agent'; not 'acted upon' by their past but freely able to make decisions about themself based on choice.

Thus behaviourism saw people as highly complex machines who could be 'programmed' or subject to positive and negative reinforcement. Psychoanalytic theory saw people as controlled by, and acting out of, their past. Humanistic theory, drawing from existential philosophy, saw people as free decision makers who could, and usually did, change according to their own wishes.

It can be argued that there are at least *two* types of humanistic psychology (Rowan, 1989; Mahrer, 1989). The first type has a particularly positive view of human beings. People, in this approach are viewed as having a tendency to 'grow' and develop. At its most extreme, this approach argues that people are essentially 'good'; an idea that dates back at least to Rousseau. It is an idea that has tended to be a reaction against the Protestant and Freudian notion of people as essentially 'evil' or bad. This 'positive' view of humanistic psychology is typified by writers such as Carl Rogers (1952; 1967) and Abraham Maslow (1972). Maslow, incidentally, is usually credited as being the person who named humanistic psychology.

The second type of humanistic psychology draws more particularly from existentialism and sees people as neither good nor bad. People, in this version are completely free. That freedom does not necessarily lead them towards goodness or badness. Essentially, then, people are 'neutral'. Representative writers of this approach include Rollo May (1989) and Erich Fromm (1975, 1979).

Humanistic psychology has as its central focus, the person. Both types acknowledge that people are complex, individual and ever changing. Thus no *one* theory of how people 'work' would necessarily explain *this* person in *this* situation. Humanistic psychology allows for this variety of human experience. It places great importance on how the individual interprets her world and does not seek to develop a 'grand theory' of how human beings think, feel and act. This is at some variance with behaviourism and psychoanalysis, both of which offer overall explanatory theories of the person.

This theme of individual, subjective interpretation or experience underpins the thinking behind the exercises in Part Two of this book. Those exercises do not tell the individual what to expect or what they *should* experience; the emphasis is on the people involved discussing what happened to them as individuals with wide varieties of thoughts, feelings, beliefs and attitudes. After all, we all come to such exercises from different backgrounds. None of our personal histories are the same.

The literature on humanistic psychology is vast (*see*, for examples Shafer, 1978; Maslow, 1972; Rowan 1988; Rowan, 1989; Wilber, 1989) and the pros and cons of this approach to psychology will not be discussed here. Suffice to say that humanistic psychology has greatly influenced both nursing and education. Carl Roger's client-centred counselling (Rogers, 1967; 1983; Burnard, 1989) has revolutionized the approach to nurse/patient relationships in psychiatric hospitals. This approach gave back to the patients their autonomy and self-direction. It was no longer nurses who made all the decisions but the patients themselves. The humanistic theme has emerged in the revised syllabi of training for general, psychiatric and mental handicap nursing.

The nursing process and nursing models also offer evidence of the impact of humanistic psychology on nursing. These models place the patient at the centre of the nursing profession and emphasize the need for individualized care planning.

Problems with the humanistic approach

All approaches to understanding the person has its problems. Humanistic psychology is no exception. First, humanistic psychology is sometimes argued to be *too* individualistic. Clearly, if everyone's experience was *completely* different to every other person's experience, communication would be impossible! It is important, therefore, to acknowledge the similarities in human experience as well as the differences. A passage attributed to the psychologist Gordon Allport sums up a useful position on this issue. All persons are, in some ways:

(a) like *all* other people,
(b) like *some* other people,
(c) like *no* other people.

Second, the 'positive' position adopted by some humanistic psychologists has sometimes been attacked as an overly optimistic one. Certainly it can be seen as a direct reaction to other, more negative, positions. As we have noted, there is an alternative position of 'neutrality'. In this position, persons are neither good nor bad: they are free to choose a whole range of behaviours. It is also arguable that 'goodness' and 'badness' are not absolutes but are social constructs. In other words, at different times in history, society dictates what passes as good or bad.

Third, humanistic psychology is sometimes viewed as having had little impact in academic circles. Carl Rogers noted in 1985 (Rogers, 1985) that it had never become a real force in psychology courses in universities. Possible reasons for this are various.

(1) It does not follow the 'scientific' traditions of behavioural psychology (and behavioural psychology has always lead the way in psychology departments in most U.K. universities).

(2) It concentrates so much on *personal* experience and not on generalisations, it is very difficult to identify particular concepts, theories and general propositions about the human situation. This makes for difficulty in establishing a formal 'knowledge base' within the field.

(3) because of the focus on the individual, traditional, quantitative research methods have not been appropriate for researching the field. Qualitative methods that suit the purpose have only recently emerged and are taking time to establish themselves as valid ones (Reason and Rowan, 1981).

In the next section, a number of humanistic themes and approaches are examined—for two reasons.

(1) The examination of these themes helps in the understanding of the concepts of both self-awareness and experiential learning.

(2) The themes under discussion are often the original sources of the exercises offered in Part Two of this book. Once again, the recurring themes will be the importance of individual interpretation of experience, the process of reflection and the value of discussion and of sharing experience.

Examples of Humanistic Influences in Experiential Learning

Co-counselling

Co-counselling is a two-way process in which two people take it in turns to spend time as 'counsellor' and 'client'. The client takes time to verbalize and talk through issues and problems from everyday life, while the counsellor gives his/her attention. Counsellors in this relationship do not act in the traditional counselling manner. In other words, they do not offer advice nor attempt to 'sort out' the client. In this self-directed approach, the clients themself learn to examine their own problems and to 'counsel themselves'. Each individual normally spends about one hour in the role of counsellor and one hour in the role of client. In this way, true interdependence is established. Neither part is wholly dependent upon the other. Responsibility is shared, though responsibility for working through problems remains firmly with the client. The counsellor may be invited to make interventions at the request of the client, according to a pre-determined contract established between them.

Co-counselling can be used in a variety of ways. It can be a means of destressing for nurses working in areas of high emotional involvement. The process of verbalizing pent-up feelings to another person in an understanding and confidential atmosphere can be very therapeutic. Co-counselling can also be used as a means of developing self-awareness through the process of exploring inner thoughts and feelings and particularly buried emotion. It can also be used as a means of practical problem solving, of talking out personal problems and making decisions about any aspects of the person's life.

Co-counselling developed in the USA under the influence of Harvey Jackins (Jackins, 1965; 1970) and, in this country, John Heron (Heron, 1974b; 1978; Heron and Reason 1981; 1982). It has made its mark within the field of experiential learning. David Potts (in Boud, 1981) has described its use as a learning tool in a university course and James Kilty (Kilty, 1982) has suggested the use of co-counselling in student nurse training. It can be of particular value as a self and peer support system for nurses working in clinical environments that are particularly stressful eg. intensive care units, children's wards, oncology departments, hospices, psychiatric units and so forth.

Co-counselling training usually takes place through a forty hour

1. People are potentially autonomous, self-directing, positive and able to exercise freedon of choice

↓

2. *However*, people are subject to a variety of stresses throughout life; early childhood experiences, partings, bereavement, difficulties in relationships, spiritual doubts and so forth

↓

3. Such stresses cause emotions (e.g. fear, anger, grief, embarrassment to become 'bottled up'

↓

4. Through talking out and through emotional relase (trembling, angry sounds, crying, laughter), those pent up emotions may be released

↓

5. Such release generates insight and enables people to think more clearly, to become less rigid, more autonomous and more able to take charge of their lives. They feel less 'acted upon' and more able to exercise choice. They can be spontaneously, positive and life asserting

↓

6. Co-counselling training, through working in pairs, offers people training in:
   (a) listening to and giving attention to others
   (b) reviewing and re-evaluating life experiences to date
   (c) the release of pent-up emotion (catharsis)
   (d) handling other people's catharsis
   (e) problem-solving and life-planning skills

Fig 2.4 *A simple map of the theory of co-counselling*

training course, during the course of one week, over two weekends or through a series of evening classes. Advanced co-counselling and co-counselling teacher training courses are also organized in colleges and extra-mural departments of universities.

Figure 2.4 is a simplified map of the theory behind co-counselling.

This is necessarily a simple guide to the theory and the reader is directed to the recommended reading list at the end of the book for a more thorough explanation of what is involved.

The assumptions behind co-counselling are that people are potentially autonomous and able to exercise choice. Through the process of living, the individual experiences various types of stress which cause the blocking or repression of emotions. If those blocked emotions can be freed, then the person can once again be capable of making life-decisions and exercising freedom of choice. Co-counselling aims at enabling individual to express that blocked feeling and thus become more able to take charge of their lives.

There are implications, here, for nursing practice. As a general rule, we usually want to calm down people who are frightened, reassure those who are crying and stop people from expressing anger. Could we as nurses be trained to *enable* people to express those emotions as a therapeutic human act? In the fields of psychiatric and mental handicap nursing, the value of such an approach is perhaps clear; expressed emotion is presumably better than repressed emotion. It is also of value in general nursing. Pre and post-operative situations, before and after childbirth, following bereavement; all these situations involve emotional experiences. Nurses can be trained to help their patients to express those feelings freely rather than a) prematurely stopping them or (b) feeling inadequate and unable to cope. Co-counselling offers one approach to coping with emotion. First, it enables the individual to experience their own emotional feelings and second, it trains people in handling other people's emotional release.

Co-counselling is a clear example of experiential learning in that it asks the individual to review past and present experience and to reconstruct their understanding in the light of the discoveries made. The co-counselling format is simple and can readily be adapted to a variety of learning situations in nurse education. A number of the exercises in Part Two of this book have been developed out of co-counselling training.

The co-counselling format can be modified in various ways. The simple pairs method can be used as an introductory activity at the start of a learning session. The group is divided into pairs and one person in each pair talks to the other about whatever is at the forefront of their mind. Their partner listens but does not comment. After five minutes, roles are reversed and the 'listener' becomes the 'talker' and *vice versa*. The pairs format can also be used to explore *particular* issues e.g. the validity of nursing models to nursing practice or the role of interpersonal skills training in nurse education—any topic that is relevant to the subject under discussion. The format offers an economical and simple method of identifying a wide range of views, thoughts, attitudes and beliefs. It also honours the *student's* views and is not heavily teacher-centred as are more traditional methods of teaching and learning.

Gestalt therapy

'Gestalt' is a German word for which there is no absolute English translation. It roughly means 'form'. Gestalt therapy, an important influence in the humanistic approach to experiential learning, is a true mind/body therapy, aiming to integrate both aspects of the person. This it does by helping the individual to become aware of both the psychological and the physiological events as they happen. Thus it has a 'here and now' focus. Gestalt therapy is only interested in the individual's past in as much as it affects a persons present-moment awareness. In an important sense, the present is all there is. The past is past and cannot be brought back, the future is yet to come and can only be speculated upon. The person who can live more fully in the present is more likely to notice, live and learn more fully.

Fritz Perls (Perls, 1969a; 1969b), a psychoanalyst, developed this approach of therapy, drawing from psychoanalysis itself, Reichian character analysis theory, existential philosophy and Eastern philosophy. By all accounts he was a charismatic character who no doubt developed his own theory in his own, idiosyncratic style. Gestalt draws from psychoanalytical theory many beliefs about 'unconscious' or unrecognized factors at work in our minds and bodies. One of its aims, like many other therapies, is to make the unconscious, conscious. It develops Reich's (1949) work on the concept of trapped emotion in the body's musculature (or what Reich called 'character armour'). Reich believed that we carry our repressed emotions around with us in our muscle clusters. Thus the person who consistently refuses to face her own anger often carries that anger around with her in the muscles of her neck and shoulders. You may want to check the status of *your own* muscle clusters and notice to what degree you continuously tense certain muscle groups. You don't? Excellent!

Gestalt is an existential approach in that it encourages the individual to take full responsibility for oneself, and acknowledges that it is *we* as individuals who invest our lives with meaning. Finally, it borrows from Eastern philosophy a fascination with paradox. Thus it is paradoxical that we often say exactly the opposite of what we really mean; e.g 'I'm perfectly relaxed' or 'It was so nice to see you again'. Again, apply this principle to yourself. How often do you say exactly the opposite of what you mean?

Perl's gestalt therapy combined all these influences to create a type of therapy that *encouraged* feelings rather than resisted them. In many other therapies, for example, the client would be helped to *oppose* their feelings. Thus the anxious person was encouraged to relax. Perl's method was to encourage the person to *experience* her anxiety and if necessary increase it. Paradoxically, as this happened, the person very often relaxed and felt more comfortable. It was through the acceptance of and experience of the emotion that release came. After all, what the anxious person is very good at doing is feeling anxious. Gestalt therapy, rather than fighting that inclination, allows it. Perl maintained that it is not until we fully accept ourselves *as we are* (and not as we would wish to be or think we ought to be) that change can come about. Further, he noted that we often blame others for our predicament ('if it wasn't for my mother ...I would be quite different) or we appeal to some dubious theory about the nature of our make up (' can't help it ...its the way I'm made!'). Gestalt therapy aims at helping the individual to experience and *own* their experiences.

As with many humanistic therapies, gestalt therapy tends to use the following 'ground rules' during practice. Gestalt therapist often prefer their clients to:

(a) Use 'I' rather than 'you', 'we' or 'people'. (Thus 'I am unhappy at the moment' rather than 'you know what it's like, you tend to get unhappy at times like this'.)

(b) Talk to others directly, in the 'first person', rather than indirectly. (Thus 'I don't agree with what you are saying' rather than 'I didn't agree with what Kevin said'.)

(c) Avoid asking questions, particularly 'why' questions. It is better to listen for the statement behind the question. Thus: 'I am hurt by what you say' rather than 'Why are you saying that?'

(d) As far as possible, remain in the present rather than slipping into reminiscences.

These ground rules are valuable in helping the individual and the group to remain fully in the present and to take responsibility for their own thoughts, feelings and actions. These ground rules are a useful set of guidelines for clear communication in *any* setting.

The gestalt therapist works by helping the client to become more aware—aware of verbal expressions, tones of voice, body movements, gestures and so forth. Such a therapist does not interpret or offer explanations of what the client is saying but encourages the client to verbalize her own insights. The aim of therapy is to increase self-awareness and self understanding through moment-to-moment observation. It encourages the person to take full responsibility for themselves, to realize that, as 'authors' of their own lives, they are free to exercise choice. In this respect, the gestalt process is similar to the co-counselling process. Both are non-interpretative and both emphasize the freedom of the individual.

The gestalt approach offers the nurse an alternative way of supporting patients. If the nurse can *allow* the patient to experience feelings—anxiety, unhappiness, loneliness as well as the more positive feelings, then (according to gestalt theory) those feelings may change. As with co-counselling, the accent is on acceptance and as with co-counselling the model is that of experiential learning; learning through direct experience.

Used skilfully, gestalt therapy is an arresting, often oblique form of dialogue which involves a wide range of techniques. Perhaps the best way to try to capture something of its variety and range is through the use of an imaginary gestalt session. In the following exchange, a nurse, Joanne, is talking to a patient, Daniel who has been admitted to an acute psychiatric unit because of his inability to cope with feelings of helplessness:

Daniel: 'There's nothing to tell really ...'
Joanne: 'Can you contradict that ...?'
Daniel: 'There's *lots* to tell ... Yes, of course that's true!'
Joanne: 'You're moving your hand in a sweeping movement ...'
Daniel: 'Yes, it reminds me of the way my father waves his arms around when he's angry ...'
Joanne: 'What would you say to your father if he were here?'
Daniel: 'I'd say: You're always angry with me-you've never given me time to talk to you.'
Joanne: 'What's your father saying back to you?'
Daniel: 'He's saying: You should grow up a bit and act your age'.

Joanne: You're smiling ...'
Daniel: Yes. I realize that there's something in what he says ...'
Joanne: 'How are you feeling now?'
Daniel: 'Sad, I suppose ... no, angry ...'
Joanne: 'Imagine that your anger was sitting in that chair, what would you say to it?'
Daniel: 'What a strange thing to ask! I'd say:'Why don't you stop messing my life up for me ...?'
Joanne: 'And what's your anger saying ...?'
Daniel: 'You never let me out ... I never see the light of day ...'
Joanne: What are you thinking ...?'
Daniel: 'I never realized before how angry I really am—with my parents ... with my whole family ... with myself ...'

And so the conversation continues with Joanne picking up the verbal and non-verbal cues that the Daniel is making explicit. No attempt is made by Joanne to interpret what Daniel says nor to offer advice. Instead, he is left to discover insights for himself and to make sense of his own experience. This imaginary conversation cannot capture the element of surprise and often relief that can occur with this type of approach. Clearly, too, training in gestalt therapy is required and training courses of various lengths are held in different parts of the country. Whilst the example, here, is from a psychiatric hospital, the gestalt approach can be used in any clinical or community setting, particularly with those people who seem to be 'stuck' with a problem or feeling. Gestalt methods can encourage new ways of looking at problems as well as generating new possible solutions.

Role Play

The use of role-play is fairly widespread in nurse education. It relates directly to psychodrama. Psychodrama was devised by the Viennese psychiatrist Jacob Moreno, who advocated the use of dramatic representations of painful, interpersonal events, played out on a stage (Moreno, 1959; 1969; 1977). His new method of therapy enabled people to try out new ways of behaving, to say things that needed saying in real life but which, in real life, were not said. In this way the person was able to rehearse new approaches to life, to try things out and to experiment. Moreno was careful to make the psychodrama realistic and even went so far as to design and build a theatre in which the psychodrama took place. In fact Moreno was the 'inventor' of many of the activities and exercises that later became widely used in self-awareness and therapy groups (Gale, 1989)

Role play as an education method emerged from this background. Role play involves the setting up of an imagined and possible situation, acting out that situation and learning from the drama. After a role play, a period of reflection is necessary, followed by feedback from other participants in order that new learning can be absorbed from the drama.

The first stage of a successful role-play, 'setting the scene', consists of inviting a number of participants to play out a scene, either from their own past or one they are likely to encounter in the future. Scenes replayed from the past are useful in that the role play allows further reflection on those past situations. Anticipated scenes, on the other hand, allow for the rehearsal of new behaviour.

Once the 'players' have been selected, scenery and props of a simple sort should be used to create the invoked scene, for example, tables and chairs, suitably arranged.

Once scenery has been set and roles cast, the role play can begin. The facilitator acts as 'director' and helps the actors to fully exploit their roles. Occasionally the facilitator may stop the role play and allow a character to slow down her acting or take time out to consider how best to play the next part of the scene.

When the scene has been played out to the satisfaction of the players, the facilitator asks the players to reflect on their performances and those of their colleagues. An appropriate feedback order is as follows:

- the principal actors self-report on their performance
- the supporting actors offer the principal actors feedback on their performance
- the audience offers the principal actors feedback on their performance
- these three stages are repeated for all the other actors
- the audience then evaluates the actor's performances and offers them feedback.

Following such feedback (which takes considerable time and should not be hurried), the role play can be re-run and new learning, gained from the feedback, can be incorporated into the new performance.

Role-play is particularly useful for teaching and learning in the following domains of interpersonal skills training:

- counselling skills training (Nelson-Jones, 1981; Burnard, 1989)
- group facilitation training (Heron, 1989b)
- assertiveness training (Alberti and Emmons, 1982; Bond, 1987)
- social skills rehearsal (Ellis and Whittington, 1981)

Apart from the use of role-play in the development of interpersonal skills, it may also be used as an aid to developing empathy; to rehearse initial practitioner/client meetings; to develop interview skills; to practice public speaking or the delivery of seminar papers and as a problem-solving activity. In this later context, a problem situation is acted out with a variety of possible 'solutions'. The actors and the audience decide which solution feels best after they have completed the various role-plays.

Figure 2.5 offers a simple map of the role-play that can be used for

Stage One:	Setting the scene; a situation or plot is decided upon.

↓

Stage Two:	Actors are selected from the group to play out various roles. Ouline 'scripts' are established.

↓

Stage Three:	The role-play is carried out.

↓

Stage Four:	Actors in the role-play evaluate their own performances and share what they have learned with the audience.

↓

Stage Five:	The audience evaluates the performaces of the actors and share what they have learned.

↓

Stage Six:	The actors are debriefed and encouraged to return to their normal selves through the use of distracting questions such as 'Can you tell me what you are planning to do this afternoon' or 'Describe the room we are sitting in.'

Fig 2.5 *A simple map of role play*

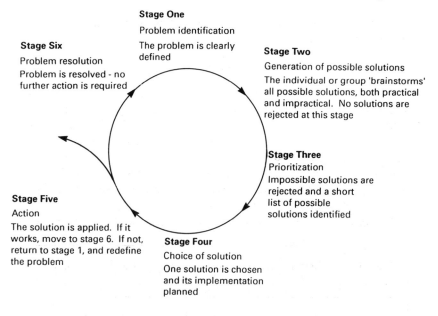

Stage One
Problem identification
The problem is clearly defined

Stage Six
Problem resolution
Problem is resolved - no further action is required

Stage Two
Generation of possible solutions
The individual or group 'brainstorms' all possible solutions, both practical and impractical. No solutions are rejected at this stage

Stage Three
Prioritization
Impossible solutions are rejected and a short list of possible solutions identified

Stage Five
Action
The solution is applied. If it works, move to stage 6. If not, return to stage 1, and redefine the problem

Stage Four
Choice of solution
One solution is chosen and its implementation planned

Fig. 2.6   *A problem-solving cycle*

setting up role-plays in a variety of educational situations. Some people love role-play: some hate it.

As with other activities in this field, participation should never be forced and only those people who *want* to take part should do so. Much can be learned vicariously by watching others engaged in role-play.

Problem Solving

The problem solving cycle (Fig 2.6) is very similar to the nursing process of the research cycle. It offers a practical and logical sequence of events for solving personal, nursing or management problems. Its use is vital as part of the process of developing the critical thinking discussed above. Such a cycle can be used by individuals on their own or by groups and is experiential in that once again it draws upon direct personal experience. It combines, too, both the learning *through* and learning *from* aspects of experiential learning. Learning through experience comes as a result of using the cycle itself and learning from experience during the 'brainstorming' phase when solutions are drawn from past experiences of problems. The term 'brainstorming' refers to the free and spontaneous generation of ideas without any attempt at censoring or filtering out less practical ideas.

The basic method of brainstorming may be described as follows. The learning group is encouraged to consider a particular topic and to call out words that they associate with it. These words are then collated on to either a black or white board or onto a series of flip-chart sheets. If the sheets are used they can be hung around the room to form a series of posters that serve as memory aids. During this initial process of the calling out of associations, the group is encouraged not to discount any association—often the more bizarre ones can lead to creative thinking (Koberg and Bagnall, 1981).

This process of encouraging associations can be a short one, taking, perhaps, up to five or ten minutes, or it can evolve into a lengthy session of up to forty minutes, as a means of investigating a topic in depth. The noting down of associations in this way can be an end in itself. The activity can lead into a discussion or a more formal lesson. In this sense, brainstorming is used as a warm-up activity to encourage initial thought about a topic.

The problem-solving cycle has many applications in the nursing field. In nurse education it may be used as a learning aid and it may also be useful as a revision aid when preparing for examinations. In the practical nursing situation it may help to identify novel ways of solving nursing problems. Nurses may also find it helpful in solving personal problems; difficulties with relationships, career changes, financial difficulties and so forth.

Meditation

Meditation, or quiet contemplation, has been advocated as a method for experiential self-discovery. It normally requires individuals to sit quietly on their own and either (a) focus their attention on one particular thought or object, or (b) merely notice and accept all thoughts and feelings as they occur, without any attempt to follow or make sense of them. Thus meditation may be active or passive.

Benson (1976), in an attempt to demystify the process of meditation noted the physiological similarities between the meditator and the person who was extremely relaxed. To this end, he preferred the term 'the relaxation response' rather than medit-ation. He advocated the use of meditation as a means of relaxation and argued that its physiological effects may be responsible for the mystical theories that have grown up around it.

The uses of meditation in the nursing field are various. Claus and Bailey (1980) edited a series of essays some of which discussed the use of meditation in preventing 'burnout' in nurses who work in stressful environments. Burnout is a feeling of apathy, dis-piritedness, physical and mental exhaustion which may occur as a result of job-related stress in the caring and teaching professions (Maslach, 1981, McIntee and Firth, 1984; Burnard, 1988). Bond and Kilty (1982) include meditation as one of their 'practical methods of coping with stress and Meg Bond discusses the value of meditation as a stress reduction method in her excellent book *Stress and Self-awareness: A Guide for Nurses*. Kilty (1982a) advocates the use of meditation in nurse education as a means of developing nurses' ability to pay attention to their patients and of developing observa-tional skills.

Meditation offers a rich and fruitful means of self-exploration and is a good experiential method of learning. It is best approached with an open mind backed up by a knowledge of possible explana-tions of the processes involved from the considerable literature on the topic. The bibliography at the end of this book includes titles on the topic and Part Two includes some meditational activities. Once learned, such procedures can easily be taught to other col-leagues and where appropriate, to patients.

Meditation as a form of experiential learning differs from other approaches discussed so far in that it tends to be solitary and introspective. It can, however, take place in the presence of others and valuable learning can take place as a result. Figure 2.7 offers a map for exploring meditation in this way. In working through the stages in this map, a form of experiential research (Reason and Rowan, 1981) is taking place. Through the sharing of personal experience, the group as a collective is developing theories about that experience that can be further tested and refined.

Stage One:	The meditation technique is decided upon and taught

↓

Stage Two:	Individual members of the group meditate for periods of between five and twenty minutes

↓

Stage Three:	On completion of the meditational period each individual describes, comments upon or 'makes sense' of the experience to the group

↓

Stage Four:	The group discusses the collective experience with a view to developing a 'theory' about what happened

↓

Stage Five:	The stages from one to four are repeated, as necessary in order to test the theory

Fig 2.7   *Meditation as a group activity*

Encounter Groups

Although the term 'encounter group' has been used in a variety of ways (Smith, 1980), it is usually traced back to the 'T' or training groups of the social psychologist, Kurt Lewin (Rowan, 1988). Lewin's T groups were not therapy groups but were designed to help managers and executives within large organizations to become more sensitive to the interpersonal and group dynamic aspects of their work (Lewin, 1952).

Ground rules, similar to those used in gestalt are often used. Schutz (1973) lists, amongst other things, the following rules for group work:

(a) Be honest with everyone, including yourself
(b) Pay close attention to what is happening in your body
(c) Concentrate on your feelings
(d) Stay with the here-and-now

(e) Take responsibility for yourself
(f) Make statements rather than ask questions
(g) Speak for yourself (use 'I' rather than 'you', 'we' or 'people')
(h) Speak directly to others.

Once again we see the familiar hallmarks of the humanistic approach to experiential learning: the personal responsibility, the accent on feelings and personal experience and the 'ownership' of those feelings.

The encounter group movement was limited largely to the United States and to the 1960's and 1970's but the effects of the movement have been pervasive. The use of structured exercises in training situation is now widespread and most people will have taken part in icebreaker exercises. These structured exercises can be of great value in the development of counselling and group skills in nurses. Through trying out new behaviours and by examining their thoughts and feelings in the supportive atmosphere of the group, nurses can develop a wide range of interpersonal skills and interpersonal competence.

The experiential learning approach: an overview

In the foregoing pages, a variety of approaches to the concept of experiential learning have been discussed. They vary in their focus and in their intention. What they all have in common is their use of human experience as the basis of learning. In the experiential learning model, learning is not a process by which facts are 'tacked on' to the person, nor is the person 'filled with knowledge'. The experiential approach acknowledges the broad and vital nature of human experience and sees it as the potential medium for fruitful learning. Figure 2.8 shows the diversity of the approach by drawing together the examples discussed so far. It will be noted, too, that the aspects of experiential learning outlined in the diagram and in the text cover all the aspects of self-awareness discussed in the previous chapter; thinking, feeling, sensing, intuiting and body experience.

Experiential Learning and the Nurse

The three elements that go to make up the concept of experiential learning are personal experience, reflection and the transformation

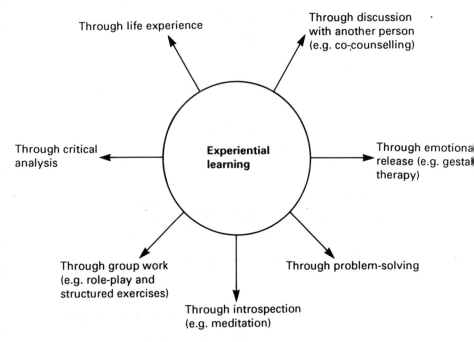

Fig. 2.8   *The variety of approaches to experiential learning*

of knowledge. There are also at least three domains in which the nurse can benefit from the experiential learning approach. These are personal growth, in general education and for the development of nursing skills Fig 2.9).

Experiential learning enhances personal growth by enabling us to develop self-awareness and to understand ourselves better. First through introspection and by receiving feedback from others we can begin to piece together more and more of the separate parts that go to make up the complex whole that we are. Second, through such methods such as group work we can explore our relationship with others. As nursing is so particularly a relationship concerned with caring for others (Morrison, 1989) it is crucial that we understand both ourselves and our abilities and weaknesses in dealing with others. Once again, we cannot begin to understand those two facets until we map out the territory, until we become aware of what we are like and how we relate to others. Armed with such awareness we are better prepared to modify our interpersonal behaviour as we see fit.

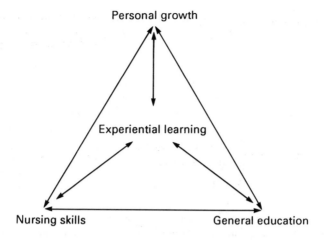

Fig. 2.9 *Experiential learning methods and the nurse*

The critical ability developed through questioning our experience can help in the domain of general education. If nursing is to continue to become a research-based profession it is vital that we arm ourselves with the necessary tools for questioning and challenging what we see and what we, ourselves, do. The reflective and critical aspects of experiential learning can help here.

Thirdly, experiential learning methods are particularly valuable in learning nursing skills, particularly the interpersonal, human skills. Thus our ability to open conversations with others comes through the *experience* of opening conversations. The skills of helping someone who is in tears develops through the *experience* of talking to someone who is crying. Conversely, being the partner of someone who is practising and developing such skills further develops our ability to relate to others. Experiential training techniques combine practice with personal experience; the chance to develop interpersonal skills through attention to the self and to others.

Next, attention is turned to the combination of experiential learning and andragogy and finally, to nurse educators' perceptions of experiential learning.

Curriculum planning in nurse education: experiential learning and andragogy

Andragogy, a term associated with Malcolm Knowles (Knowles, 1978; 1980; 1984), though used before his time, is one used to differentiate the theory and practice of adult education from pedagogy—the theory and practice of the education of children. Knowles claimed that adults differed in some fundamental ways from children and, therefore, required a different educational system. Such a system included the ideas that:

● adult education should be grounded in the participants wealth of prior experience
● adults need to be able to apply what they learn
● adult education should be an active rather than a passive process.

All of these ideas have much in common with the concept of experiential learning described here. Out of these ideas, Knowles drew up a method of conducting adult education sessions.

One objection that may be raised about Knowles' theory is that the ideas identified above may be applicable, also, to children. If this is the case, it is difficult to see how he can argue for a discreet theory of adult education based on these principles. Knowles acknowledges this problem and, in later writing, tends to describe andragogy as an attitude towards education rather than as being a discreet theory of adult education. This argument and others relating to andragogy have been well described by Jarvis (1983, 1984) and Brookfield (1987).

Andragogy has much in common with the student-centred learning approach of the late Carl Rogers (1983). This is not surprising as both Knowles and Rogers were influenced, through their respective professors of education, by John Dewey, the pragmatist and philosopher of education (Dewey, 1966; 1971; Kirschenbaum, 1979). It also has much in common with many of the approaches to experiential learning, emphasizing, as they do, the centrality of personal experience and subjective interpretation.

How, then, may aspects of experiential learning and andragogy usefully be combined in nurse education? Such a combination needs to take into account certain basic principles such as negotiation, the importance of personal experience and the use of self and peer assessment. What must also be borne in mind, however, is that learner nurses and nurse educators have to work to a prescribed syllabus of training laid down by the English and Welsh National

Boards even if such syllabi are *interpreted* by individual schools and colleges. This fact makes nurse education somewhat different to many of the experiential learning training workshops at where all of the content may arise out of the participants needs and wants. Many nurse educators may encounter problems in translating workshop experience into practice because of this fact. Also, there is a large difference between using experiential learning methods in a two-day to one-week training workshop and using them on a regular basis throughout a three year programme.

Figure 2.10 offers a tentative cycle which acknowledges both the principles of andragogy and the principles of experiential learning, as outlined in this chapter.

In stage one, two things happen. First, the students identify their own learning needs through direction from the tutor and in line with the 'learning contract' approach described by Knowles (1975). Second, the tutor identifies certain learning needs out of the pre-scribed syllabus. The students can draw from their previous ward experience, here, and may find a 'brainstorming' session a useful means of generating topics.

Thus, in stage two, a timetable is negotiated. It will consist of the two elements described above and may be divided into a 'theory' element and a 'skills' element. The skills element may include both practical nursing skills and interpersonal skills, as appropriate. Again, it will be remembered that the content of this theory and skills mix will arise jointly out of the expressed needs of the students and the suggested ideas of the nurse tutor.

The theory element may then be learned using a whole range of educational approaches, including the traditional ones of lecture and seminar, as required. However, for the skills element, it is recommended that the experiential learning cycle be followed.

The cycle, briefly outlined here incorporates the student-cen-tred, negotiating approach of andragogy with the accent on personal experience and self and peer evaluation of experiential learning. It also acknowledges that learner nurses need to work to a syllabus and that nurse educators can contribute much to effectively planning a course of study around such a syllabus. In this cycle, 'negotiation' means just that—the programme emerges out of the experience and knowledge of both students and tutors.

The approach offers a balance between what Heron (1986) calls 'following' and 'leading'. Following involves taking the lead from the students, using their experience and ideas. Leading, on the other

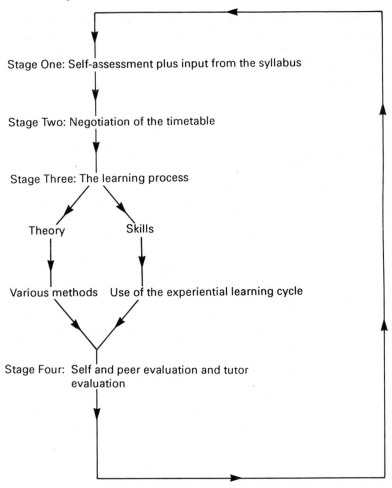

Stage One: Self-assessment plus input from the syllabus

Stage Two: Negotiation of the timetable

Stage Three: The learning process

Theory   Skills

Various methods   Use of the experiential learning cycle

Stage Four: Self and peer evaluation and tutor
evaluation

Fig. 2.10   *A cycle for combining andragogy and experiential learning in nurse education*

hand, means making suggestions and using structure to help the
students. Together, these methods can ensure balance and symmetry in the nurse education programme. If the programme involves too much 'following' or is too student-directed in its methods,
it will be unbalanced. On the other hand, if it involves too much
'leading' or is too teacher-directed in its methods, it will also be
unbalanced.

Having said this, the attitude towards nurse education should always remain student centred. The issue is not whether or not the tutor or the student should serve as the focal point of the educational process but the means by which the students educational needs are identified and satisfied. In this sense, then, the focus remains the student.

Nurse educators' perceptions of experiential learning

Nurse educators are perhaps the people who use experiential learning methods more than anyone. Given that the experiential learning approach is a relatively new one in nurse education, it was decided to explore nurse educators perceptions of experiential learning (Burnard, 1989c). Twelve nurse educators from different parts of the U.K. and all of whom claimed to use experiential learning methods were interviewed using a semi-structured interview approach. The interviews were transcribed and a modified 'grounded theory' approach (Glasser and Strauss, 1967) was used to explore and categorize the data. The following headings and subheadings emerged. They are offered, here, as a series of lists to enable the reader to sample the sorts of issues that some educators are discussing when they turn to the topic of experiential learning. A fuller report of this part of the study is offered elsewhere (Burnard, 1989). The headings of the categories of response are turned into questions, for the sake of clarity. It is stressed that this does not necessarily mean that those questions were posed so formally in the interviews.

The categories and sub categories gleaned from the interview transcripts are as follows: the responses under each heading are in rank order (i.e. the first response was the most frequently cited one, the last was the least frequently cited.)

What is experiential learning?
● learning through doing
● affective learning
● whole life experience
● learning from present experience
● role-play.

What are experiential learning methods?

- reflective activities
- role-play
- practical activities (including clinical work)
- structured group activities
- humanistic therapies
- games and simulations
- altered states of consciousness
- use of T.V.'s, computers and videos,
- physical activities.

What are the advantages of experiential learning approaches?

- they are useful for teaching interpersonal skills
- experiential learning increases self-awareness
- they are 'real/whole/active'
- they are lighthearted and fun
- I enjoy using them
- they are a more relaxed approach to learning
- they are useful for teaching practical nursing skills
- they are easier to use than other methods.

What are the disadvantages of experiential learning approaches?

- They can be uncomfortable or threatening for the students
- They are not suitable for all topics on the syllabus
- They need lots of planning
- They are time consuming
- Transfer of learning may be a problem.

How do you evaluate experiential learning?

- Through verbal feedback from the group
- By written reports from the students
- Through repertory grid techniques
- Via written reports from the clinical areas
- Through personal observation.

Student nurses perceptions of experiential learning

In the second stage of the research project briefly outlined above, 12 student nurses from various parts of the UK were interviewed and the transcripts of their interviews analysed in using the grounded theory approach. Their responses (and the categories generated out of their interviews) were different to those of the nurse educators.

The categories and sub categories gleaned from the interview transcripts are as follows: the responses under each heading are in rank order (i.e. the first response was the most frequently cited one, the last was the least frequently cited).

What is experiential learning?

- learning through doing
- 'practice' rather than 'theory'
- it is not textbook learning
- it involves a set of exercises used in the school of nursing
- learning in the clinical setting
- it does not involve 'chalk and talk' teaching
- it is the whole of life experience.

What are your thoughts abut experiential learning in the clinical setting?

- clinical learning is better than school learning
- school learning is not necessarily linked with clinical learning
- clinical learning is 'real'.

What experiential learning activities have you take part in the school of nursing?

- role play
- small group work
- empathy building activities
- clinical skills development
- 'blind walk'
- psychodrama
- counselling skills activities
- icebreakers.

What are the advantages of experiential learning activities?

- they offer the chance to learn from personal experience
- they can develop interpersonal skills
- they are an aid to learning
- they are enjoyable
- they are an aid to reflection.

What are the disadvantages of experiential learning activities?

- they can be unreal
- they don't suit all learners
- they can be threatening
- they can be silly or embarrassing
- 'I don't like role play'
- they could get out of control.

It is interesting to compare the two sets of responses. It is not intended that those responses be discussed in detail, here: they are offered as examples of how two groups of people perceived experiential learning. It is repeated that the responses were offered freely and not in response to the *questions* displayed above. Those questions are used as *category headings* to group together responses from the transcripts. Overall, it is notable that the students tended to view clinical work as an example of experiential learning far more readily than did the nurse educators. It is notable, too, that the two groups seem to make a distinction that Boud (1989) makes, between experiential learning as:

(a) what people are engaged in and value as a process of learning, and
(b) a set of activities that educators use.

It would seem that the students in this study are often trying to describe what they see as valuable and useful in experiential learning and the educators are describing what they *do*. It is also notable that the students tended to be more critical of the experiential learning approach than did the educators. This research is ongoing.

A Case in Point: One

Sarah, a tutor in a school of nursing in a large general hospital planned a course in counselling skills for second and third year students as part of their core curriculum. She planned a series of ten one day workshops spread throughout the second year with more to follow in the third. The decision was made to use the first two study days to introduce the general approach and method of teaching and learning.

The first study day was a disaster. The students didn't understand what was happening and didn't understand why they were being to take part in the 'odd' exercises. One student said she hadn't learnt anything at all. Two said they enjoyed it and would like more. The rest were fairly non commital.

After a change of plan, Sarah used the second study day to explain the *principles* of experiential and adult learning. She explained the rationale behind the use of group activities and exercises and asked the students to temporarily suspend judgement on what they were asked to take part in.

Gradually, the students took to the approach and by the end of the first two months, most were enjoying the study days. All of them said that they helped in their clinical work and had relevance. Some students remained wary of the methods used but most enjoyed the first year. Sarah decided to use the first study days with the *next* set of students to work through the principles of the approach. She realized that she had tried to rush the use of experiential learning methods and the 'slope' at which she had introduced them had been too steep.

Experiential learning in North America: a personal viewpoint

Given that the experiential learning approach developed out of the educational system prevalent in the USA and that most of the key figures in the development of experiential learning theory were American, it was decided to study the use of experiential learning methods in nurse education in Canada and the USA (Burnard, 1987). Two months were spent in various parts of Canada and the USA, including Edmonton and Calgary in Canada and San Francisco, Florida, the New York/New Jersey area and Boston visiting various colleges and university departments that were responsible for the education and training of nurses. Certain key themes developed out of these visits and are offered here as a subjective picture of one person's view of some aspects of interpersonal skills training in North America. Clearly, given the size, variety and cultural difference to the U.K., another commentator would observe other things and draw other conclusions.

The first observation was that nursing programmes in North America appear to have a very high *theoretical* component. This seems to have lead to the learning process becoming very *teacher centred*. There seemed to be little time for developing student-centred methods in initial nurse training given this emphasis on a large theoretical input.

Nursing courses in North America are generally very carefully pre-planned and pre-programmed. Often students were armed with very detailed programmes of aims and objectives, learning goals, reading lists and lecture times. There seemed little space for negotiation and all students tended to follow a similar course to their colleagues. There seemed to be little opportunity for individualizing courses to suit individual students.

When experiential learning methods such as role-play, small group discussion, process recording and video recording *were* used, they were used very skilfully and professionally. They were often used to teach counselling skills and basic clinical skills. Some hospitals and colleges were equipped with fully laid out mock ups of wards, complete with double mirrors and video recording equipment which students could use to monitor and develop their skills. It was notable that American students were generally less frightened of video equipment than is the case with some UK students. They also tended to be more likely to 'open up' in discussion and to express their point of view more assertively.

Overall, the impression was that experiential learning methods were not used to direct a *whole course* nor were they used in the intimate, small group manner that they are often used in schools and colleges in the UK. Clearly, part of this is due to the far larger numbers of students being admitted to courses in North America than is generally the case in the U.K. More usually, experiential learning methods were used as specific 'training' techniques and these were often extremely well planned activities that had very clear learning objectives and very definite stages to be worked through. The 'learning to objectives' model seems to be very prevalent in parts of North America and this may not be surprising given the accent on the acquisition of so much knowledge. Sometimes (and particularly on the West Coast), the experiential learning approach was associated with the 1960's 'encounter group' movement. On the east coast, the prevailing psychological model often seemed to be a psychodynamic one and thus the humanistic approach was not so prevalent.

Often, it seemed as though American people generally and nurses particularly, were more socially skilled than is the case in the UK. Clearly this is linked to certain cultural differences. It was notable, for instance, that people were often much more at ease with handling introductions, discussions and farewells. Whether or not this is due to any particular training methods or whether it is part of the American culture is hard to say.

Overall, the feeling was that experiential learning methods, despite the fact that (in the literature at least) they had developed in the USA, were not particularly widely used. It is always difficult to make such sweeping generalizations about somewhere as vast as North America and it is fully acknowledged that there are bound to be places were a fully experiential model *is* used. Often, more interactive and experiential learning methods were used in Master's degree courses which many nurses now see as part of their essential education and training in the USA.

These, then, are some impressions of the use of experiential learning methods in the USA. It will be interesting to see the degree to which, with Project 2000 and the movement of nursing education in the UK towards colleges and universities, UK nursing education moves more towards the American style of education.

Conclusion

This chapter has explored the concept of experiential learning from a variety of points of view. It started by noting the variety of definitions that have been used in the literature. It then explored aspects of the concept that seem common to *all* approaches to experiential learning. Humanistic and other themes common in the experiential learning approach were discussed and practical issues explored. Finally, a brief reference to research and to the American situation were made. In the section that follows, these themes are translated into practice through the offering of ranges of experiential learning activities for the development of counselling and group skills. Self-awareness continues as a necessary prerequisite of all skilful human intervention.

In closing this chapter, it is important to consider the question of training for experiential learning facilitation. David Boud sums up the problems in this area well:

> One of the questions that arises is how sophisticated should training be? Too often those working in experiential education are simply doing what they have picked up as an adjunct to their normal work. They have learned from experience but their experience is limited. There is little training available and, sometimes, desired. However, unless we are challenged to move beyond our existing practices then experiential education will remain forever peripheral to mainstream education and promise more than it can deliver (Boud 1989)

Boud was not writing, particularly, about nurse educators and nurse education. But he might have been. The challenge must be to incorporate experiential learning methods into mainstream nurse education so that they are less the domain of a few, interested people, but are available to all.

A Case in Point: Two

Peter had been using experiential learning methods for a number of years, in a college responsible for running post registration courses for nurses. All of the courses that he offered were 'experiential' in nature and he gradually came to use less and less structure and to offer less and less theory inputs to course members. He felt that it was important to listen to the students and to respond to their expressed wants and needs. He often told his colleagues that 'traditional' lecturers worried far too much about 'knowledge' and not enough about skills and 'process'.

In one course evaluation, he was distressed to find out that he had gained a reputation, not for teaching or for learning but for 'doing therapy'. He discovered that many nurses were worried about his study days and tried to avoid attending them. There were reports that 'you have to disclose everything' on his courses. After considerable discussion with his friends and colleagues, he decided to reintroduce more structure and achieved a balance between both process and content. He also tried his hand at one or two straight lectures and found that he enjoyed giving them. Gradually, he worked out a style of working that involved experiential learning, information giving and negotiation with the students.

PART TWO

LEARNING SKILLS THROUGH EXPERIENCE

3

Using Experiential Learning Activities

> We learn through experience and experiencing, and no one teaches us anything. If the environment permits it, anyone can learn what he chooses to learn; and if the individual permits, the environment will teach everything it has to teach (Spolin. 1963).

This chapter offers concrete guidance on the use of the exercises for interpersonal skills development offered in the next three chapters. Each exercise is laid out under a series of headings, as follows:

Aim of the activity

Here, the intention of the activity is made clear. What can never be written for such exercises is a series of behavioural objectives. As we have noted throughout this book, experiential learning is necessarily idiosyncratic. It is not possible to predict the outcome of a particular exercise for any particular person. All that can be said is that there is a clear intention in setting out to offer the exercise as a learning activity. On the other hand, it is important not to be too wide-eyed an innocent about this. Once the facilitators have used these activities a number of times, they will come to recognize certain typical patterns of response. These can help in shaping future courses and in the development of new activities and exercises.

Number of participants recommended

Whilst a minimum and maximum figure is quoted for each activity, many of the activities can be adapted for larger numbers. Many, too, can be carried out by only two persons, learning as a pair. If larger numbers are being catered for, it is important that a great deal of structure is used in organizing the exercise. In groups of 20 and above, it is helpful if the instructions for the activity are written out in the form of a pre-prepared handout, so that everyone is clear about how to proceed. It is also helpful if, during the feedback and processing session, the larger group is broken up into smaller groups of about four or five people. Many do not like discussing their experience in a large group and constraints of time may mean that not everyone gets heard in a larger group. A chairperson may be nominated or elected in each feedback group. A short plenary session with the whole group may be facilitated afterwards as a means of maintaining group cohesion.

Environmental considerations

The usual suggestion, here, is that group members sit round in a circle. Such a circle is symbolic of unity and also ensures that the group facilitator is on an equal footing with the group and not physically (and symbolically) set apart from it. It is important, too, that the group does not sit around a table or in front of desks. In this way, there are no physical barriers between participants. The arrangement also allows for greater ease of movement if the exercise calls for the group's splitting into pairs or smaller groups.

Equipment Required

None of the exercises calls for equipment difficult to obtain. The most important feature of the exercises is the personal one; the meeting of people to enhance their skills.

Time required

Taking time over these activities is very important. None of them should be rushed and plenty of time should be allowed for the discussional part of the activity. If the activities take significantly shorter time to complete than is suggested in the text, it is worth reflecting on what parts you are hurrying. The most frequently rushed part of the activities is the *reflective* part, when group members reconvene and discuss what happened. This is a shame as it is this reflective and discussionary period which is the most important of the whole activity. So ...take your time!

The process

This section, in each case, offers a clear, stage by stage account of how to run the exercise. Initially it is useful if these instructions are followed to the letter. Once the facilitator and the group have become familiar with the approach, various modifications can be made to suit the circumstances. Many of the most effective activities are those that the facilitators devise themselves. On the other hand, as was noted above, it is important that none of the exercises is rushed.

Evaluation

This section offers questions that the facilitator may want to ask of the group. They are meant as guidelines only. Clearly, the questions that arise out of the process of the group activity are far more useful than any preconceived ones. It is hoped, though, that the questions in these sections stimulate ideas for your own questions.

Notes

Sometimes there are variations on an activity that can be used in different situations that can be used to explore different aspects of interpersonal skills. These notes offer suggestions for such variations and, sometimes, lead the way to further reading.

Using the activities

A useful procedure for planning the use of these exercises is outlined in Fig 3.1, an experiential learning plan. Example programmes for teaching counselling skills and for teaching group facilitation skills are also offered at the ends of the next two chapters.

In the cycle in Fig 3.1, a short theory input is offered if the exercise is to be used in a classroom. If it is to be used in a peer learning group, a discussion or reading period may be substituted for this stage. The theory input should be kept fairly short and to the point and should not become a full-blown lecture. The aim of such a theory input is to set the scene and to offer a minimal theoretical framework through which students can test some of their experiences.

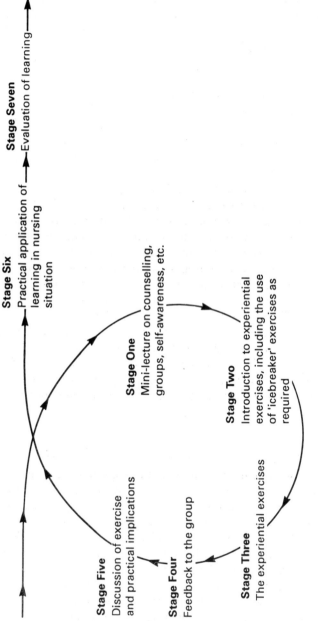

Stage Seven
Evaluation of learning

Stage Six
Practical application of
learning in nursing
situation

Stage One
Mini-lecture on counselling,
groups, self-awareness, etc.

Stage Two
Introduction to experiential
exercises, including the use
of 'icebreaker' exercises as
required

Stage Three
The experiential exercises

Stage Four
Feedback to the group

Stage Five
Discussion of exercise
and practical implications

Fig. 3.1   *Experiential learning cycle for nurses*

Second, the aim of the experiential exercise is introduced to the group. It seems reasonable to tell the students what you have in mind when you ask them to undertake an activity, although there are problems here too. If you are *too* explicit about your aims, you stand to limit the student's own perceptions of what they experience. They will be looking to satisfy your aim. On the other hand, to suggest that you have *no* aim in mind, seems naive if not dishonest! No one suggests an activity for no reason at all!

Third, the exercise is carried out as outlined. Following the exercise, all participants feedback their experiences to each other and to the group. Out of this feed back can be developed a fruitful discussion and the learning that has taken place may become the basis for practical use in the 'real' nursing situation.

Finally, the learning is applied and the nurse carries his or her new skills into the clinical area or into the community. This is the crucial test of the experiential learning method: that skills are transferred from the classroom to the clinical setting. *How* this occurs is fraught. One way of encouraging such transfer is for tutors and lecturers to ensure that nurses receive sufficient clinical support and to ensure that they, as teachers of the skills, are seen in the clinical areas as credible role models as well as teachers.

The experiential learning cycle can be evaluated through further discussion at a later date and further repetitions of the learning cycle carried out. The learning cycle, then, combines experiential learning from the clinical setting with experiential learning in the school or college and back again. The stages are now described in more detail.

Stage One

The mini-lecture or theory input should be a short theoretical exposition of the particular topic being explored. The aim, as we have seen, should be to create a theoretical framework through which students can make sense of their coming experience. There is no reason why such a theory input has to be given by the facilitator. It is often better given by a student or by a group of students. A useful method is to break the student group up into smaller sub groups and invite each of the sub groups to research and give a short input on one aspect of the topic. What is to be avoided at all costs, however, is students reading lengthy papers on the topic. A short series of headings and one or two main references will often suffice. It is probably better to underteach than to overteach.

Stage Two

A concept of experiential learning is introduced briefly and clearly. Any questions about the nature of the exercises are answered in a straightforward manner and students are offered the option of either taking part or observing their colleagues. One of the aims of this part of the session should be the 'demystifying' of the students. Students have often been socialized into fairly traditional expectations of what teachers and learners do. To suddenly overwhelm them with activity based learning is not a good plan. Nor is the 'try it and see' approach; students are generally more comfortable if they know a little of what to expect in advance.

Before the exercises are carried out, it is sometimes of value to use one or more 'icebreaker'. Icebreakers are short activities carried out by the group which serve to create a relaxed and open atmosphere in which group members can enter more fully into the exercise being undertaken. A selection of such exercises are describe here; others may be found in a number of publications listed at the end of this book. Most are lighthearted and should be treated as such. Ice-breakers similar to or variants of these activities can be found in a variety of sources (see, for example Heron, 1973; Pfeiffer and Jones, 1974; Kilty, 1982a).

Opinions about the use and appropriateness of icebreakers vary. Some people like using them and some loathe their use. Some students enjoy them and find them helpful, others find them embarrassing. My own experience is that younger people, for what-ever reasons, find them easier and more helpful than do older people. The general rule here perhaps, is to try them and see what happens. If the group that you are working with don't like them, start sessions off in another way.

Some facilitators use icebreakers as a form of introductory activity with new groups of students or at the beginning of a workshop. Another format for such introductions is as follows:

The facilitator invites each person, in turn, to identify the following things about themselves:

- their name (or the name they prefer to be known by)
- their current job
- three things about themselves that are unconnected with work.

Alternatively, the group can be divided up into pairs and the members of the pairs interview each other. After about ten minutes, each of the pairs return to the group and each person is introduced to the group, by her partner.

Icebreakers

1. Milling and pairing

Group members move around the room. At a signal from the facilitator they stop and pair off with their nearest colleague. The pairs spend a few minutes sharing thoughts on one of the following:

(a) a recent pleasant experience
(b) two interests away from work
(c) feelings about the group or about the workshop.

2. Mirroring

Group members wander around the room and periodically stop in front of each other. When they do so, each pair attempts to mirror the body position and facial expression of the other.

3. Sculpture

Group member pair off. One member then moves the other into any position that he or she chooses, as a shop dummy might be moved. The group member being sculpted in this way stays in the position that she has be put in. The 'sculptors' then wander around and view each others work.

4. A Piece of music ...a book ...

The facilitator asks each member in turn to describe herself in the following ways:

(a) 'If you were a piece of music, what would you be? Describe yourself as that.
(b) If your were a book, what book would you be? Describe yourself as that.
(c) If you were a building, what building would you be? Describe yourself as that.

5. Compliments

Group members complete a 'round' in which they turn to the person on their left and complete the sentence:

'What I like most about you is ...'

Other sentences that can be used here include:
'I imagine that you are ...'
'I would like to be like you for this reason ...'
'I appreciate ...'

6. Awareness

Group members complete a 'round' in which they turn to the person on the left and complete the sentence:'Now I am aware of ...'. They complete the sentence by noticing something about the person sitting on their left. Group members are encouraged not to rehearse their responses but to respond spontaneously as their turn comes.

7. Formative experiences

Group members recall three formative experiences from their lives to date and share those experiences with the group. The experiences should be positive ones.

Some of these icebreakers will be easier to carry out and take part in than others. Much will depend on how well group members know each other. If a lighthearted, open manner is adopted by the facilitator, many people will find them easy, amusing and sometimes revealing. Others will not and no one should be forced to take part in an icebreaking activity that they are not happy to undertake.

Stage three

In this stage, the experiential learning exercises described in the following chapters are carried out.

Stage four

Following the exercise, group members are invited to feedback their experiences of the exercise. Usually a broad open question such as

'What happened?' will be sufficient to encourage people to share what happened during the activity. It is important that each member is allowed to contribute as hear she sees fit and is 'heard'. On the other hand, it is not the facilitators role to make sure that *everyone* has a say. A participants choice to say nothing should be respected.

This stage of the cycle should be as lengthy as necessary to ensure that all that needs to be shared *is* shared. It is probably during this reflective phase that most new learning occurs. This is equivalent to part of the 'transformation of knowledge' phase of Kolb's learning cycle, discussed in Chapter 2.

Stage five

During the fifth stage, new learning from the shared experience is applied in a practical way. Group members discuss the application of what has been learned to the clinical or community nursing situation. Thus, if a counselling exercise has been carried out to develop listening skills, the group considers ways in which the nurses present could use their new listening skills to enhance patient care. Sometimes it can be helpful if psychodrama or role-play is used here, to rehearse the process of using the particular skill. It is useful, too, if group members undertake to try out a new skill the day that it is learned—away from the group. In this way the new learning is reinforced, becomes more real and is better remembered. There is a great danger of experiential learning activities producing skills that are then not transferred to the clinical situation. The experiential learning session becomes an interesting but historic 'island' in group members memories.

Stage six

This stage, the stage of practical application, takes place away from the classroom. It is the stage in which theory is transformed into practice and in which the new human skills are practised. It is a time of trial and error but also of discovery. It is a time of testing out 'what worked in the learning session' against 'what happens in the clinical setting'. If the gap between the two is too great, then the temptation will always be to slip back to old patterns of behaviour that worked in the past. Application of new learning takes courage and it is here that students will need plenty of clinical support.

Self-monitoring is essential in this stage and it helps if students are encouraged to keep a journal or diary. A modified version of the journal format, described here, has been used at the School of Nursing Studies, University of Wales College of Medicine, as part of a continuous assessment procedure during the Bachelor of Nursing course, during student's psychiatric nursing secondment. It has met with varying amounts of success. After an initial period of the students' feeling that they would not be able to complete the journal, a number found it particularly useful and planned to continue to use it throughout other parts of their course. Others continued to find it difficult to use and one never completed it.

The instructions for completion of the journal are simple. Participants are required to make weekly entries in a suitable book under the following headings:

- Problems encountered and how they were resolved
- How new skills were applied
- New skills required to be learned
- Personal growth issues/self awareness development
- Other comments.

These headings can be varied according to the needs and wants of a particular group using the journal approach. No guidelines need to be given regarding the amount that is written under each heading. The finished product need not be an 'academic' piece but should be a free representation of the student's experience.

Group members are encouraged to make regular entries and this regularity tends to make the process of keeping the diary easier. Participants who try to 'catch up' and complete the whole thing in one last go tend to have difficulty in remembering what has happened and generally the process is less valuable.

Stage seven

Stage seven is the stage of evaluation of both the experiential learning and of the practical application of that learning. Depending on how you define 'experiential learning', it may be argued that *both* of these two aspects are examples of experiential learning; there is the learning from the group and the learning from practical experience. The following is a useful format for carrying our such an evaluation:

1. Each group member gives feedback on (a) the negative and (b) the positive aspects of his or her performance. It is important that this order is observed so that the individual ends her own self-evaluation on a positive note.

2. The group member who has thus self-evaluated invites comments from the group and the tutor or lecturer, again on the negative and then the positive aspects of his or her performance. This will only apply if colleagues of the teacher have been actively involved with that person during their time in the clinical setting.

An alternative method, as we have noted above, is to use the dairy or journal as the basis of self-evaluation. This can be done in one of two ways:

(a) The person meets with his or her tutor or lecturer and discusses his or her diary with the educator or

(b) The person meets with his or her peer group and all of the diaries and all of the experiences are discussed in a group setting. Out of this group meeting can emerge the general aims of the next learning session.

These processes incorporate both self and peer evaluation. Such a combination is valuable in that it encourages both reflection by the individual on her own performance and feedback from others. Luft, (1967) argues that both self-disclosure and feedback from others are the two vital ingredients for self awareness.

If self and peer evaluation are two aspects of feedback to students, then the third element is feedback from the tutor/lecturer or sister/charge nurse. If three reports of a given person are obtained in this way, 'triangulation' has taken place (Fig 3.2). Hopefully, the student receives an important mixture of both subjective and objective evaluation data.

Continuing the cycle

Once a round of the cycle has been complete, the learning gained can be carried forward into a new cycle. Nurse education and training programmes using a module scheme can incorporate the experiential learning cycle into curriculum plans to create a continuous cycle of experience, reflection, learning and application, thus operationalizing experiential learning theory.

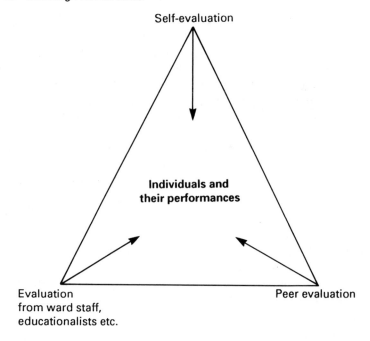

Fig. 3.2 *Triangulation in the evaluation process*

The next chapters describe a series of experiential exercises that may be used to develop human skills; (a) in the one-to-one interpersonal relationship (counselling skills) and (b) in the one-to-group relationship (group and facilitation styles). The final chapter offers a number of exercises for the development of self awareness; awareness that can enhance both counselling and group skills.

4

Experiential Exercises for Human Skills—Counselling Skills

> Life is a voyage in which we choose neither vessel nor
> weather, but much can be done in the management
> of the sails and the guidance of the helm (Petty, 1962).

Counselling may be described as a therapeutic conversation between two people in an understanding atmosphere. The breadth
of such a definition is intentional and aimed to cover a whole
range of situations which may be described as 'counselling'. Consider, for example, the following:

● talking to a person who is about to undergo an operation and who is
  confused and upset
● discussing progress in the clinical situation with a student nurse
● helping a colleague to reach a decision about a career change.

Arguably, all of these situations are counselling situations. The
skills that are often associated with professional counsellors are also
those that are required by the professional nurse.

Personal qualities of the nurse as counsellor

Counselling in nursing requires at least two things: (a) the development of certain personal qualities and (b) the learning of basic interpersonal skills. Three clusters of personal qualities identified by
humanistic therapist and educator Carl Rogers (1967, 1983) as necessary for an effective therapeutic relationship were:

(1) Warmth and genuineness
(2) Empathic understanding and
(3) Unconditional positive regard.

The three clusters of qualities are now briefly described and related to nursing.

Warmth and genuineness

Warmth, in the nursing relationship refers to being approachable and open to the patient or colleague. Schulman (1982) argues that the following characteristics are involved in demonstrating the concept of warmth; equal worth, absence of blame, nondefensiveness and closeness. Warmth is as much a frame of mind as a skill and perhaps one developed through being honest with yourself and being prepared to be open with others. It also involves treating the other person as an equal human being.

Martin Buber (1958) the philosopher and therapist made a distinction between the 'I-it' relationship and the 'I-thou (or 'I-you') relationship. In the I-it relationship, one person treats the other as an object, as a thing. In the I-thou relationship, there occurs a meeting of persons, transcending any differences there may be in terms of status, background, lifestyle, belief or value systems. In the I-thou relationship there is a sense sharing and of mutuality, a sense that can be contagious and is of particular value in nursing.

What is not clear is the degree to which a nurse-patient relationship can be a mutual relationship. Rogers (1967) argues that the relationship *can* be a mutual one but Buber acknowledges that because it is always the client who seeks out the professional and comes to that professional with problems, the relationship is, necessarily, unequal and lacking in mutuality. For Buber, the professional relationship starts and progresses from an unequal footing:

> He comes for help to you. You don't come for help to him. And not only this, but you are able, more or less to help him ... You are, of course, a very important person for him. But not a person whom he wants to see and to know and is able to. He is floundering around, he comes to you. He is, may I say, entangled in your life, in your thoughts, in your being, your communication, and so on. But he is not interested in you as you. It cannot be. (Buber 1965).

Thus warmth must be offered by the nurse but the feeling may not necessarily be reciprocated by the client. There is, as well, another problem with the notion of warmth. We all perceive personal qualities in different sorts of ways. One person's warmth is another person's sickliness or sentimentality. We cannot guarantee how our 'warmth' will be perceived by the other person. In a more general way, however, 'warmth' may be compared to 'coldness'. It is clear that the 'cold' person would not be the ideal person to undertake helping another person in a nursing setting! It is salutary, however, to reflect on the degree to which there are 'cold' people working in the nursing arena and to question why this may be so. It is possible that interpersonal skills training may help this situation for it may be that some 'cold' people are unaware of their coldness.

To a degree, however, our relationships with others tend to be self-monitoring. To a degree, we anticipate, as we go on with a relationship, the effect we are having on others and modify our presentation of self accordingly. Thus we soon get to know if our 'warmth' is too much for the patient or colleague or is being perceived by him in a negative way. This ability to constantly monitor ourselves and our relationships is an important part of the process of developing interpersonal and counselling skills.

Genuineness, too, is another important aspect of the relationship. In one sense, the issue is black or white. We either genuinely care for the person in front of us or we do not. We cannot easily fake professional interest. We must be interested. Some people, however, will interest us more than others. Often, those clients who remind us of our own problems or our own personalities will interest us most of all. This is not so important as our having a genuine interest in the fact that the relationship is happening at all.

On the surface of it, there may appear to be a conflict between the concept of genuineness and the self-monitoring alluded to above. Self-monitoring may be thought of as 'artificial' or contrived and therefore not genuine. The 'genuineness', discussed here, relates to the nursing professional's interest in the human relationship that is developing between the two people. Any way in which that relationship can be enhanced must serve a valuable purpose. It is quite possible to be 'genuine' and yet aware of what is happening: genuine and yet committed to increasing interpersonal competence.

Empathic understanding

> 'First of all,' he said, 'if you can learn a simple trick Scout, you'll get along a lot better with all kinds of folks. You never really understand a person until you consider things from his point of view ...'
> 'Sir?'
> '... until you climb into his skin and walk around in it.' (Lee, 1960).

Empathy is a relatively new term, apparently coined by Titchner in 1909 to translate the German term 'Einfuhlung' (Bateson and

---

A Case in Point: Three

A college of nursing in the south of England planned its new nursing curriculum along experiential lines. Students were to be encouraged to negotiate their learning needs with the tutors and lecturers and most learning sessions were to include activities and exercises. Evaluation was to include not only the whether or not the students had learned but also feedback to teachers on their style of facilitation.

Mary has been a nurse tutor for sixteen years and was nearing retirement. She was suddenly deskilled by the new approach and preferred a style of teaching which allowed her more control over lessons and did not involve the 'soul searching' of the experiential learning approach. Whilst some of the younger members of the teaching team were disparaging about her, the principal was able to appreciate the need for flexibility in curriculum planning and worked out a series of teaching session with Mary that made full use of her skills, whilst not forcing her to adapt to activity based teaching and learning.

Coke, 1981). The term is usually used to convey the idea of the ability to enter the perceptual world of the other person; to see the world as they see it. It also suggests an ability to convey this perception to the other person. Kalisch (1971) defines empathy as 'the ability to perceive accurately the feelings of another person and to communicate this understanding to him'.

Empathy is different to sympathy. Sympathy suggests 'feeling sorry' for the other person or, perhaps, identifying with how they feel. If a person sympathizes they imagine themselves as being in the other person's position. With empathy the person tries to imagine how it is to be the other person. Feeling sorry for that person does not really come into it. Being empathic, says Rogers:

> ... means entering the private perceptual world of
> the other and becoming thoroughly at home in it. It
> involves being sensitive, moment to moment, to the
> changing felt meanings which flow in this other
> person, to the fear or rage or tenderness or confusion
> or whatever ... (Rogers, 1967)

The process of developing empathy involves something of an act of faith. When we empathize with another person, we cannot know what the outcome of that empathizing will be. If we pre-empt the outcome of our empathizing, we are already not empathizing—we are thinking of solutions and of ways of influencing the client towards a particular goal that we have in mind. The process of empathizing involves entering into the perceptual world of the other person without necessarily knowing where that process will lead to.

Developing empathic understanding is the process of exploring the client's world, with the client, neither judging nor necessarily offering advice. Perhaps it can be achieved best through the process of carefully attending and listening to the other person and, perhaps, by use of the skills known as 'reflection' which is discussed in a later chapter of this book. It is also a 'way of being', a disposition towards the client, a willingness to explore the other person's problems and to allow the other person to express themselves fully. Again, as with all aspects of the 'client-centred' approach to caring, the empathic approach is underpinned by the idea that it is the client, in the end, who will find their own way through and will find their own answers to their problems in living. To be empathic is to be a fellow traveller, a friend to the person as they undertake the search. Empathic understanding, then, invokes the notion of 'befriending'.

There are, of course, limitations to the degree to which we can truly empathize. Because we all live in different 'worlds' based on our particular culture, education, physiology, belief systems and so forth, we all view that world slightly differently. Thus, to truly empathize with another person would involve actually becoming that other person! We can, however, strive to get as close to the perceptual world of the other by listening and attending and by suspending judgement. We can also learn to forget ourselves, temporarily and give ourselves as completely as we can to the other person. There is an interesting paradox involved here. First, we need self-awareness to enable us to develop empathy. Then we need to forget ourselves in order to truly give our empathic attention to the other person.

Unconditional positive regard

Carl Roger's phrase 'unconditional positive regard' (Rogers 1967), conveys a particularly important predisposition towards the client, by the nurse. Rogers also called it 'prizing' or even just 'accepting'. It means that the client is viewed with dignity and valued as a worthwhile and positive human being. The 'unconditional' prefix refers to the idea that such regard is offered without any preconditions.

Often in relationships, some sort of reciprocity is demanded: I will like you (or love you) as long as you return that liking or loving. Rogers is asking that the feelings that the nursing professional holds for the client should be undemanding and not requiring reciprocation.

There is a suggestion of an inherent 'goodness' within the client, bound up in Roger's notion of unconditional positive regard. This notion of persons as essentially good can be traced back, at least to Rousseau's 'Emile' and is philosophically problematic. Arguably, notions such as 'goodness' and 'badness' are social constructions and to argue that a person is born good or bad is fraught. However, as a practical starting point in the nursing relationship, it seems to be a good idea that we assume an inherent, positive and life-asserting characteristic in the client. It seems difficult to argue otherwise. It would be odd, for instance, to engage in the process of counselling with the view that the person was essentially bad, negative and unlikely to grow or develop!

Unconditional positive regard, then, involves a deep and positive feeling for the other person, perhaps equivalent, in the health professions to what Alistair Campbell has called 'moderated love' (Campbell 1984). He talks of 'lovers and professors', suggesting that certain professionals profess to love, thus claiming both the ability to be professional and to express altruistic love or disinterested love for others. It is interesting that Campbell seems to be suggesting that a nursing professional can 'professionally care' or even 'professionally love' her client.

These, then, are the personal qualities that are an important aspect of the counselling relationship. An interesting question is the degree to which such personal qualities can be *learned*. It is perhaps likely that most of us start off with a disposition towards such qualities and that such a disposition can be enhanced by the person paying attention to developing it. Certainly, counselling can never be an automatic, machine-like process. We cannot simply turn on our counselling skills.

On the other hand, neither can we only depend upon having the required personal qualities. If that were so, a lot of people would never even attempt to be nurses or counsellors! The secret lies, perhaps, in combining personal qualities with certain, definable counselling skills. It is here, however that another paradox lies. Can we develop usable counselling skills that we have practised in the presence of our colleagues and friends and still maintain a

Stage One:	Individuals are unaware of the range of interpersonal and counselling skills available to them. If they do encounter such a range, they are likely to see the use of such frameworks as 'unnatural' or 'artificial'. This is the person who will argue that counsellors and communicators are born rather than made.

↓

Stage Two:	Individuals attending a course or a workshop and explore a range of counselling skills. At this point, because they are *thinking* about what they are doing in their relationships with others, they temporarily become clumsy and awkward.

↓

Stage Three:	Individuals have come to incorporate the new skills into their own repertoire. The person is both 'skilled' and 'natural'.

Fig 4.1:   *A three stage model of the development of interpersonal and counselling skills*

naturalness and spontaneity—a personal style? Certainly we can. It is worth considering, for a moment, a three stage model of interpersonal or counselling skills training (Fig 4.1).

The model is fairly self-explanatory. The person who is new to interpersonal and counselling skills training may be threatened or dismissive of it. As people come to learn more about such training, they begin to experiment with new skills and temporarily becomes *deskilled*. As they progress, they gradually incorporate the new skills into their own personal style. People are no longer awkward nor a clone of other people. They have developed their own therapeutic style.

Counselling Skills in Nursing

It is helpful to divide the skills of counselling into two groups:

(a) Listening and attending and
(b) Counselling interventions.

The exercises described in this chapter are aimed at developing both of these groups of skills. The exercises may be worked through systematically or individual exercises may be singled out to explore a particular skill.

In order to place these two groups of skills in context, a map of the counselling process is offered in Fig 4.2. In stage one, the counsellor and client meet and gradually come to know each other. This stage may be seen as paralleling the first stage of the nurse/patient relationship. Often it is a thawing out process for both the counsellor (or the nurse) and the client (or the patient).

As the counsellor/client or nurse/patient relationship develops the client slowly tests the boundaries of the relationship through discussion of safe, surface issues. Then as trust develops, the topic slowly shifts to deeper existential issues (or to the person's 'deeper' problems). At this stage, the client often realizes the depth of feeling that he or she has about particular issues: emotional release may occur through the shedding of tears, the expression of anger or through embarrassed laughter. Such a release is known as catharsis and the counsellor or nurse can develop the skills required in helping a person through the process of cathartic release. Such release or catharsis often enables the client to develop new insights into their condition. It is as though the tears or anger clear away a veil which covers possible solutions to problems or new ways of looking at life issues. Reflection on those new insights can lead to problem solving and future planning. Such a stage is an important one. Cathartic release, on its own, is not sufficient. Counselling, if it is to help, must be a practical activity. Therefore, the person being counselled needs to be able to plan out what they will do with the insights gained from the emotional release.

Once plans have been made, perhaps through the medium of the counselling or nursing relationship, the client will want to act on those plans. Thus, stage 7, the action stage, takes place away from the counsellor/client relationship and in the client's life situation. Problems, in the end, are not solved by sitting and talking but rather by action. It is the relationship prior to this action that has enabled the action to occur. During this stage, the counsellor's role may only be a supportive one.

Finally, as the client develops more and more autonomy and self-direction, he or she will need the help of the counsellor or nurse less and less. The time comes when the counselling relationship needs to be terminated and the client and counsellor part. This

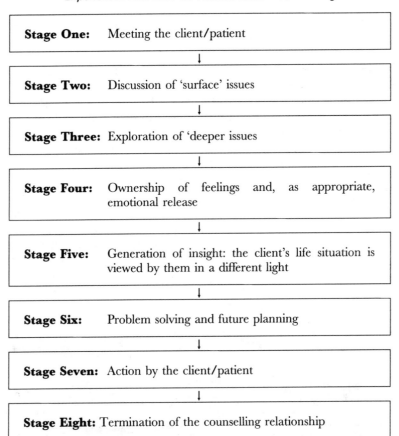

Stage One:	Meeting the client/patient
Stage Two:	Discussion of 'surface' issues
Stage Three:	Exploration of 'deeper issues
Stage Four:	Ownership of feelings and, as appropriate, emotional release
Stage Five:	Generation of insight: the client's life situation is viewed by them in a different light
Stage Six:	Problem solving and future planning
Stage Seven:	Action by the client/patient
Stage Eight:	Termination of the counselling relationship

Fig. 4.2   *A map of the counselling process*

will often raise all sorts of issues about dependency and independence both in the counsellor and the client. The nurse who is undertaking a lot of counselling needs to explore how he or she feels about partings and about saying goodbye. Stop reading for a moment and consider what it would feel like to say goodbye to someone close to you. Notice the thoughts and feelings that are brought to the surface by such an idea. Now consider what it may be like for clients who have spent a fair amount of time sharing themself with another person and getting to know that person well. Consider, now, how best you can handle such situations, both from the point of view of *you* as counsellor and of the client.

The map of events described here is an over simplification. Human relationships are rarely as clear-cut as this. The map does however offer some signposts for the direction that the counselling relationship may take. All the stages in the map are also stages in the nurse/patient relationship, although the depth of that relationship will depend upon the needs of the particular patient and the skills of the particular nurse. It is worth bearing in mind that it should always be the client or patient who determines the rate at which the relationship develops. It is, after all, the *client or patient's relationship*. It is not the counsellor or nurses role to probe, interrogate or in any way force disclosure. Such disclosure, if it is to be therapeutic must be offered freely by the client or patient and with their goodwill.

The skills described here are ones that can be useful in a wide range of nursing situations from helping the bereaved person, to counselling colleagues and friends to helping people who have just received bad news.

Listening and attending

To listen to another person is the most human of actions. In counselling it is the crucial skill. The experiential exercises that follow aim to develop the skill of listening and giving attention. Listening refers to the process of *hearing* what the client is saying. Hearing encompasses not only the words that are being used but also the non-verbal aspects of the encounter. Thus *attending* refers to the counsellor's skill in paying attention to the client, in keeping attention focused 'out' as described in the first chapter.

Throughout all the exercises in this chapter, the words facilitator, counsellor and client are used for convenience. It should be noted that the words tutor (or lecturer), nurse and patient can just as easily be used in their place.

Once again, the participants in these exercises are exhorted to 'stay awake' whilst doing them. It is vital that people *notice* their own feelings and thoughts, his own body position, posture, eye contact and so forth. The mystic, George Gurdjieff, maintained that for most of what we call the waking state, we were, in fact, 'asleep'—we simply do not *notice* (Reyner, 1984). Ouspensky, a follower of Gurdjieff went on to suggest that we only really learned new things and remembered what was happening to us when we 'stayed awake'. The Christian mystic, Simone Weil added a spiritual dimension to the notion of attending when she suggested that true noticing of what was happening around us was an acknowledgement of God (Weill 1967). Brother Lawrence called noticing and attending 'The Practice of the Presence of God' (Lawrence 1981). Thus the topic has been addressed both from secular and spiritual points of view.

The nurse who practices regularly the feat of noticing can become more observant, more sensitive to the needs of others and more self-aware, Indeed, to notice in this way is to be fully present in the moment that is being lived. The first series of exercises concentrates on a variety of aspects of listening and attending.

Exercise 1

Aim of the exercise: To enable participants to get attention 'out'.
Group Size: Any number from 6 to 20
Time Required: About 20 to 30 minutes.
Materials and/or Environment Required: A large, comfortable room and a circle of straight-backed chairs.

Process

1. The facilitator invites the group to divide into pairs.
2. Each pair nominates one of them as 'A' and one as 'B'.
3. 'A' then describes in detail for two minutes, what 'B' looks like; hair, facial expression, clothing and so on. Such a description should be 'literal' and concrete and free of value judgements.
4. 'B' listens silently to 'A''s description.
5. After five minutes the facilitator invites the pairs to exchange roles: thus 'B' describes, literally, 'A's appearance.
6. When both aspects of the exercise have been completed, the facilitator asks the group to reconvene and encourages feedback with an open question such as 'What happened?'

Evaluation

The facilitator may also want to explore with the group how they *felt* about doing the exercise. He or she may also encourage group members to describe any problems that they have with the activity.

Notes

A 'solo' version of this activity can be used as a method of paying attention to and describing a person (or an object) outside of oneself as a method of getting attention 'out' prior to talking to a patient or commencing counselling. In this case, it is done silently and alone and is valuable as a means of freshening attention at any time.

Exercise 2

Aim of the Exercise: To explore proximity and spatial relationships between two people.
Group Size: Any number from 6 to 20.
Time Required: About 1 hour.
Materials and/or Environment Required: A large, comfortable room and a circle of straight-backed chairs.

Process

1. The facilitator ask the group to divide into pairs.
2. Each pair nominates one of them as 'A' and the other as 'B'.
3. 'A' and 'B' then sit about four feet apart and hold a conversation.
4. After five minutes, 'A' and 'B' move their seats forward until their knees are almost touching and continue the conversation for another five minutes.
5. After the second phase of the activity, the facilitator leads a discussion on the issue of space between talker and listener.

Evaluation

The facilitator may want to ask:

- Which was worse, sitting too close or too far away?
- Do you ever stand or sit to close to other people?

Notes

On the subject of proximity, Roger Brown (1965) makes the interesting observation that you can move someone backwards round a room by constantly overstepping the 'right' space between you, by small increments! A curious fact. Try it!

It is important to discuss *cultural* differences in acceptable spaces between people. This is a vital issue when counselling people from different cultures.

Exercise 3

Aim of the Exercise: To explore eye contact whilst listening.
Group size: Any number from 6 to 20.
Time required: About 1 hour.
Materials and/or environment required: A large, comfortable room and a circle of straight-backed chairs.

Process

1. The facilitator invites the group to divide into pairs.
2. Each pair nominates one of them as 'A' and one as 'B'.
3. 'A' talks to 'B' on one of the following topics:
   (a) favourite foods
   (b) people I like
   (c) why I want to stay in nursing.
4. During this time, 'A' tries to maintain *constant* eye contact.
5. After five minutes, 'A' and 'B' switch roles and 'A' talks to 'B' whilst 'B' maintains *constant* eye contact.

Evaluation

The facilitator may want to ask:

● What did that feel like?
● How do you *know* how much eye contact to make?
● What makes eye contact difficult?

Notes

The notes, above, about cultural factors apply equally much to the issue of eye contact. It is easy to mismanage the question of eye contact where people from very different cultures are concerned.

Exercise 4

Aim of the Exercise: To explore the verbal and non-verbal aspects of listening.
Group size: Any number from 6 to 20.
Time required: About 40 minutes.
Materials and/or environment required: A large, comfortable room and a circle of straight-backed chairs.

Process

1. The facilitator invites the group to divide into pairs.
2. Each pair nominates one of them as 'A' and on as 'B'.
3. 'A' talks to 'B' for five minutes on one of the following topics:
    (a) interests away from work,
    (b) recent clinical experiences,
    (c) past or future holidays.
4. Whilst 'A' is talking, 'B' does *not* listen.
5. After five minutes, the facilitator asks the pairs to exchange roles: thus 'B' talks to 'A' and 'A' does not listen.
6. When both aspects of the exercise have been completed, the facilitator invites the group to reconvene and encourages feedback with an open question.

Evaluation

The facilitator may want to explore the following sorts of questions with the group:

- What did it feel like *not* to be listened to?
- What did it feel like to sit and *not* listen to someone?
- What did you do to *avoid* listening?
- What did you do when you realised you could hear what the other person was saying?
- Do you recognise the 'non-listener' from clinical practice?
- How effective is *your* listening ability?

Notes

A variation on this exercise is to have the pairs sitting back-to back, so that 'A' talks to 'B' but cannot see 'B'.

Effective Listening Behaviours

Following this exercise it is common for a discussion to develop on the importance of non-verbal behaviour when listening to another person or when counselling them. Gerard Egan (1982) offers a useful acronym for remembering the important aspects of non-verbal activity during the listening process. This is illustrated in Fig. 4.3.

Egan argues that, in Western countries, these behaviours are usually associated with effective listening. Sitting squarely means sitting opposite the person who is being listened too, rather than next to them. In this way, the one doing the listening can see *all* of the other person and can observe the non-verbal behaviours of the talker. The position also demonstrates interest in the other person.

An open position means that the listener does not have his or her arms crossed. Such crossings can be create real or psychological barriers. The *closed* position can often be construed as being defensive, as we shall see in the next exercise.

Eye contact should be steady and appropriate. No one wants to be stared at but neither do they want to feel that the person who is supposed to be listening to them will look anywhere but at them. As we have noted, too, cultural factors play a part in determining how much or how little eye contact may be made. Eye contact may also depend upon the relative status of the pair involved. Finally, the listener should try to sit quietly and be relaxed. T.S. Eliot summed up this position well when he wrote:

> 'Teach us to care and not to care.
> Teach us to sit still.' (Eliot, 1963).

When listening to another person, we do not have to be constantly rehearsing what *we* will say next. Nor do we have to relate everything that is said to *us* and to our own thoughts and feelings. The ability to sit and quietly listen may be the greatest of all counselling skills.

S —Sit *squarely* in relation to the person.
O—Maintain an *open* position.
L —*Lean* slightly towards the other person.
E —Maintain reasonable *eye contact* with them.
R —Try to *relax*.

Fig. 4.3 *The behavioural aspects of listening (after Egan 1982)*

Egan's guidelines on how to sit when listening to another person may be useful as a baseline. Clearly, no one wants to talk to a person who sits and looks like a statue! On the other hand, it doesn't help very much to sit, lounge and fidget when listening. The SOLER acronym serves as a gentle reminder and guide whilst listening and counselling. Don't become a slave to it.

Exercise 5

Aim of the Exercise: To explore the verbal and non-verbal aspects of listening and giving attention.
Group Size: Any number from 6 to 20.
Time Required: About 40 minutes.
Materials and/or environment required: A large, comfortable room and a circle of straight-backed chairs.

Process

1. The facilitator asks the group to divide into pairs.
2. Each pair nominates one of them as 'A' and one as 'B'.
3. 'A' talks to 'B' for five minutes on one of the following topics:
   (a) the future of nursing
   (b) problems of training
   (c) music and/or books that I like
4. 'B' *contradicts* the first four SOLER behaviours described in the text. In other words, she:
   (a) does *not* sit squarely to the other person but sits next to her instead,
   (b) maintains a *closed* position with arms and legs crossed,
   (c) leans *away* from the other person, rather than *towards* him,
   (d) makes *no* eye contact with the other person ... BUT *listens to 'A'*!
5. After five minutes, roles are reversed and 'B' talks to 'A', whilst 'A' contradicts the first four SOLER behaviours.
6. When both aspects of the exercises have been completed, the facilitator convenes a remeeting of the group and leads a discussion about what happened.

Evaluation

The facilitator may want to ask:

- What did it feel like to be listened to by someone who *did not appear* to be listening to you?
- What was it like *not* to demonstrate that you were listening?
- What does all this say about your own listening?

Notes

The facilitator is advised to suggest to the group that they do not overdramatize the contradictions of the SOLER behaviours and also to emphasize the fact that group members are to listen to each other. This last fact tends to get forgotten when the behaviours are contradicted!

Minimal Prompts

For this and other exercises, group members may find the use of 'minimal prompts' helpful. Figure 4.4 offers examples of such prompts. The aim is to become familiar with the range of possible prompts available and to use them knowingly and out of choice. Often our behaviour becomes so automatic that we do not notice the

Examples of Verbal Prompts
'Yes'
'O.K.'
'Go on ...'
'Ah-ha'
'Mm ...'
'Right'
'I see ...'
Examples of Non-verbal Prompts
Head nods
Smiles
Raised eyebrows
Encouraging hand movements
Gentle touch

Fig. 4.4   *Examples of minimal prompts in listening*

minimal prompts that we use in everyday conversation. Exercises of this sort can help to encourage people to make conscious decisions about their use of such prompts.

Exercise 6

Aim of the exercise: To explore the use of minimal prompts.
Group size: Any number from 6 to 20.
Time required: About 40 minutes to 1 hour.
Materials and/or environment required: A large, comfortable room and a circle of straight-backed chairs.

Process

1. The facilitator invites the group to divide into pairs.
2. Each pair nominates one of them as 'A' and one as 'B'.
3. 'A' talks to 'B' for five minutes about one of the following topics:
    (a) the sort of person that I would like to be
    (b) my skills as a nurse
    (c) what I would do if I had a million pounds.
4. 'B' listens but uses *exaggerated* minimal prompts and does not talk or respond the 'B' in any other way.
5. After five minutes, roles are reversed and 'B' talks to 'A', whilst 'A' uses exaggerated minimal prompts.
6. When both parts of the exercise have been completed, the group is reconvened and the facilitator leads a discussion on what happened.

Evaluation

The facilitator may like to ask the group:

● What were you reminded of when you did this exercise?
● Are you ever *normally* like this?
● Were you reminded of anyone else when you did this activity?
● What are the problems of overuse of minimal prompts?

Notes

This exercise is an example of what may be called exaggerated negative role play. Practising *poor* examples of counselling skills can be a powerful way of encouraging *good* practice. Activities of this sort can cause much hilarity on the part of the participants!

Exercise 7

Aim of the exercise: To practice listening and giving attention with appropriate verbal and non-verbal behaviours.
Group size: Any number from 6 to 20.
Time required: About 1 hour.
Materials and/or environment required: A large, comfortable room and a circle of straight-backed chairs.

Process

1. The facilitator asks the group to divide into pairs,
2. Each pair nominates one of them as 'A' and one as 'B.'
3. 'A' talks to 'B' for five minutes about one of the following topics:
   (a) the house/flat that I live in
   (b) my family
   (c) my political beliefs
4. 'B' listens to 'A' and observes the SOLER behaviours. Thus she:
   (a) sits squarely
   (b) maintains an open position
   (c) leans slightly towards to the other person
   (d) maintains steady and comfortable eye contact
   (e) relaxes.

   'B' may also use minimal prompts but uses them sparingly and consciously.
5. After five minutes, roles are reversed and 'B' talks to 'A' for five minutes whilst 'A' maintains the SOLER behaviours and uses appropriate minimal prompts.
6. When both aspects of the exercise have been completed, the group is reconvened and the facilitator leads a discussion on what happened.

Evaluation

The facilitator may want to ask the group:

- Was this better or worse that the previous exercise?
- What was it like to be listened too?
- What was it like to listen to the other person?

Notes

It is important that the facilitator emphasises that this is not a conversation. The listeners should restrict themselves to minimal prompts and not respond in any other way to what their partners say.

It is possible to experiment with the exaggerated negative role-play, described above. Using this approach, group members are encouraged to try out using the SOLER behaviours in an exaggerated way. It is advised, however, that the negative approach is used sparingly and not as a routine part of interpersonal skills training. In fact it is important that *no* aspects of interpersonal skills training become routine. The secret, here, is to continuously modify your approach. If, as a trainer, you find yourself getting into a rut, it is likely that the people in your groups will be getting into one too.

Exercise 8

Aim of the exercise: To reinforce the skills of listening and attending with appropriate verbal and non-verbal behaviours.
Group size: Any number from 6 to 20
Time required: About 1–1½ hour.
Materials and/or environment required: A large, comfortable room and a circle of straight-backed chairs.

Process

1. The facilitator asks the group to divide into threes.
2. The threes are invited to nominate 'A', 'B' and 'C'.
3. 'B' talks to 'B' for five minutes on any topic.
4. 'B' listens to 'A' and uses the SOLER behaviours and minimal prompts in an appropriate manner.

5. 'C' acts as a process observer and makes notes on 'B''s perform-ance as a listener.
6. After five minutes, each trio feeds back to itself in the following order:
   (a) listeners describe their own performance,
   (b) talkers describe the listeners' behaviour,
   (c) process observers describe the listeners' behaviour.
   In each case, it is only the listener's performance that is under discussion.
7. After ten minutes, 'A', 'B' and 'C' exchange roles and the exercise is repeated. The same assessment procedure is used after the repeat.
8. When all participants have been in the roles of listener, talker and process observer, the facilitator invites the group to reconvene and encourages feedback on the activity.

Notes

The trio's feedback procedure is a vital part of the process of this activity and should not be skipped or rushed. It represents the 'reflection' period of the experiential learning cycle described in earlier chapters. The order of the feedback encourages self-evaluation followed by peer-evaluation.

Exercise 9

Aim of the exercise: To test the effectiveness of the listening and attending exercises.
Group size: Any number from 6 to 20.
Time required: About 1–1½ hours.
Materials and/or environment required: A large, comfort-able room and a circle of straight-backed chairs.

Process

1. The facilitator asks the group to divide into pairs.
2. Each pair nominates one of them as 'A' and one as 'B'.
3. 'A' talks to 'B' for three periods of three minutes on any topic.

1. 'A' talks to 'B' for three minutes
2. 'B' paraphrases what 'A' has said
3. 'A' talks for a further three minutes
4. 'B' paraphrases what 'A' has said
5. 'A' talks to 'B' for a final three minutes
6. 'B' paraphrases what 'A' has said

Fig. 4.5   *The order of exercise 9*

4. 'B' listens to 'A' whilst observing the SOLER behaviours and using appropriate minimal prompts.
5. *Between* each three minute period, 'B' paraphrases what 'A' has said, to 'A''s satisfaction. The order is made clear in Fig 4.5.
6. After the cycle has been completed, 'A' and 'B' exchange roles and complete stage 5, above.
7. When the entire cycle has been completed, the facilitator reconvenes the group and invites feedback.

Evaluation

The facilitator may find it useful to ask the following questions:

● What problems did you have with paraphrasing?
● Were all the talkers satisfied with the paraphrasing?
● Could you use paraphrasing in counselling?
● If so, when?

Notes

This exercise can also be used with process observers. Such an observer can be allocated to each pair. Feedback in each trio then takes place as follows:

(a) the listener feedsback on her or her own performance,
(b) the talker offers feedback to the listener,
(c) the process observer offers the listener feedback.

Once again, the only feedback is to the listener as the aim of the exercise is to encourage and develop listening skills. This exercise further enhances self-monitoring, self assessment and peer evaluation. A form of this exercise was originally used by Carl Rogers

Places I have visited.
What I admire in others.
How I feel about myself.
Common problems I experience in the clinical setting.
What I intend to be doing in five years time.
What I did before I came into nursing.
My family.
My views about marriage.
My spiritual beliefs (or lack of them).
What I would do if I wasn't a nurse.
My views on recent news events.
How I feel about 'green' issues.
How I cope with stress.
How I feel about nursing.
Caring for the elderly.
What I was like as a child.
What I would be like if I was a member of the opposite sex.
How other people see me.
How my parents see me.
A period of history that I would like to have lived through.
Things that make me angry.
Things I like about myself.

Fig. 4.6 *Topics for use in attending and listening exercises*

(Kirschenbaum, 1979) as a method of developing client-centred counselling skills.

Figure 4.6 offers a range of topics that can be used for any of the attending and listening skills exercises described in this section. Sometimes, however, it is best to either a) determine the topics according to current areas of debate within the group or b) allow group members to decide on their own topics. Group members should always be encouraged to *be themselves* in these exercises and not to act out a particular role. This personalises the learning that takes place and ensures that the exercises develop skills that can transfer back to the clinical setting.

Exercise 10

Aim of the exercise: To explore the groups need to improve their listening skills.

Group size: any number from 6 to 20.
Time Required: About 20–40 minutes, depending on the size of the group.
Materials and/or environment required: A large, comfortable room and a circle of straight-backed chairs.

Process

1. Each person in turn, completes the statement: 'What I need to do to improve my skills as a listener is ...'. Each group member can complete the statement in any way he or she chooses.
2. When each person has contributed, the facilitator encourages a discussion about improving listening skills.

Evaluation: The facilitator may like to ask the group:

- What did it feel like to wait your turn in this exercise?
- What similarities and differences are their between group members?
- How *will* people improve their listening skills?

Notes:

There are various other statements that can be used in place of the one offered above. Examples include:

- Situations in which I find it difficult to listen include ...
- I don't always listen very well because ...
- I would be a better listener if ...
- If I was a better listener I would ...

Counselling Interventions

The bases of effective counselling are the skills of listening and giving attention. Second to these comes the need to use effective verbal interventions. A format for understanding the range of useful and therapeutic interventions has been devised by John Heron (Heron 1989a) and is called *Six Category Intervention Analysis*.

This conceptual framework was developed by Heron out of the work of Blake and Mouton (1976). It was offered as a conceptual model for understanding interpersonal relationships, and as an assessment tool for identifying a range of possible therapeutic interactions between two people.

The Category	What the counsellor/nurse does
Authoritative interventions	
1. Prescriptive	Makes suggestions, recommends behaviours, offers advice.
2. Informative	Gives new knowledge or information.
3. Confronting	Challenges what the other person says or does.
Facilitative interventions	
4. Cathartic	Helps the other person to release pent up feelings and emotions.
5. Catalytic	Helps to 'draw out' the other person.
6. Supportive	Encourages and affirms the worth of the other person.

Fig. 4.7 *The six categories of therapeutic intervention (after Heron 1989a)*

The six categories in Heron's analysis are: prescriptive (offering advice), informative (offering information), confronting (challenging), cathartic (enabling the expression of pent-up emotions), catalytic ('drawing out') and supportive (confirming or encouraging) (See Fig 4.7). The word 'intervention' is used to describe any statement that the practitioner may use. The word 'category' is used to denote a range of related interventions.

Heron (1989a) calls the first three categories of intervention, (prescriptive, informative and confronting), 'authoritative' and suggests that in using these categories the practitioner retains control over the relationship. He calls the second three categories of intervention (cathartic, catalytic and supportive), 'facilitative' and suggests that these enable the client to retain control over the relationship. In other words, the first three are 'practitioner-centred' and the second three are 'client-centred'. Another way of describing the difference between the first and second sets of three categories is that the first three are 'You tell me' interventions and the second three are 'I tell you' interventions.

What, then, is the value of such an analysis of therapeutic interventions? First, it identifies the *range* of possible interventions available to the nurse/counsellor. Very often, in day to day interactions with others, we stick to repetitive forms of conversation and response simply because we are not aware that other options are available to us. This analysis identifies an exhaustive range of types of human interventions. Second, by identifying the sorts of interventions we can use, we can act more precisely and with a greater sense of intention. The nurse/patient relationship thus becomes more particular and less haphazard; we know *what* we are saying and also *how* we are saying it. We have greater interpersonal choice.

Third, the analysis offers an instrument for training. Once the categories have been identified, they can be used for students and others to identify their weaknesses and strengths across the interpersonal spectrum. Nurses can, in this way, develop a wide and comprehensive range of interpersonal skills.

It is worth repeating that the skills identified in this chapter as counselling skills are exactly similar to the basic human skills used in day to day nursing interactions. Thus an understanding of the full range of the six categories can enhance and enrich the quality of the nurse's approach to care. It should be noted, too, that the analysis does not offer a mechanical approach to interpersonal skills training. The exercises here will not simply be a training in learning particular phrases and reposes. This is an important issue. The analysis indicates a *type* of response. The choice of words, the tone of voice, the non-verbal aspects of a particular response must develop out of the individual's belief and value system and out of their life experience. Those aspects of the response are also dependent upon the situation at the time and upon the people involved. All human relationships occur within a particular context. It is impossible to identify what will necessarily be the right thing to do in *this* situation at *this* time. A mechanical, learning-by-heart approach to counselling or interpersonal skills would, therefore, be inappropriate. In the descriptions of the following exercises, examples are offered but when the exercises are carried out, each student will have to find his own words, his own expressions and his own personal approach. This affirms the basic principle of human skills training; the honouring of personal experience developed through observation and reflection.

Nurses' perceptions of their interpersonal skills

In two recent studies, we invited both student nurses and trained nursing staff to identify their own strengths and weaknesses in terms of the *Six Category Intervention Analysis* (Burnard and Morrison, 1988; Morrison and Burnard, 1989). In the first study, using an accidental sample of 92 trained nurses, those nurses were asked to rank order the six categories according to how skilful they thought they were in using them. Generally speaking the nurses perceived themselves to be more skilled in using the authoritative categories and less skilled in using the facilitative categories. Having said that, *most* of the nurses perceived themselves as being particularly weak in using *cathartic* and *catalytic* interventions. Overall, they perceived themselves as being best at being supportive.

There were marked similarities in the findings of the second study in which we invited 84 student nurses to rank order the six categories in terms of their perceived strengths and weaknesses in using them. Again we found an overall picture of greater perceived skill in using authoritative interventions rather than facilitative ones. Students also thought that they were generally most effective in using supportive interventions and not so good at using cathartic and confronting interventions. In general, the results of both studies support Heron's (1989a) assertion that a wide range of practitioners in our society show a much greater deficit in the skilful use of facilitative interventions that they do in the skilful use of authoritative ones.

Using the exercises

Two principles should be observed when using the exercises in this section. Participation in them should always be voluntary. Growth in interpersonal development can never be enhanced if participation is enforced. This, then, is the *voluntary principle*. The other principle is the *gymnasium principle* (Heron, 1977b). Just as a gymnast exercises one of muscles in isolation to the rest that would not normally be used in that way, so the exercises that follow pick out one small aspect of the counselling relationship. Just as the gymnast later feels the benefit of exercising different sets of muscles, so nurses feel more interpersonally competent when they have undertaken the whole range of activities described here. The learning from particular exercises needs to be incorporated into everyday life just as the gymnast needs to use all his muscles in day to day living.

Figure 4.8 offers some examples of interventions within the six categories. It must be repeated, however, that the important issue is that such interventions develop naturally out of the context the nurse and patient find themselves in. The examples are offered

ı. Prescriptive	(a)	'Perhaps you would like to talk to your family about this.'
	(b)	'I suggest you talk to your GP about the rash.'
2. Informative	(a)	'These tablets may make you feel a bit drowsy.'
	(b)	'There is a *Relate* office in .....'
3. Confronting	(a)	'We agreed to stop at 3pm, so we will stop now.'
	(b)	'I notice that you very frequently talk about how much you hate your husband and you also say that you will stay with him ...'
4. Cathartic	(a)	'Its all right with me if you want to cry.'
	(b)	'What do you *really* want to say now..?'
5. Catalytic	(a)	'Can you say more ...?
	(b)	'What happened then?
6. Supportive	(a)	'I appreciate your being here.'
	(b)	'I enjoy spending time with you.'

Fig. 4.8   *Examples of interventions within the six categories*

only as a means of clarifying the concept of the six categories and not as exemplars or as 'ideal types'.

In a more general sense, the six categories of intervention have a wider application, beyond the counselling relationship. The nurse working in a hospice, for example, may need considerable cathartic skills in order to enable the expression of feelings. The charge nurse will require prescriptive skills when delegating ward duties. All nurses require the ability to be appropriately supportive. Nurse educators will find that the whole range of interventions can be used in the contexts of teaching and learning. Indeed the process of experiential learning is particularly facilitated by the skilful use of the cathartic, catalytic and supportive categories.

There may be situations in which skilful use of a *particular* category may be required in this way. The nurse who is skilled in all six categories can deftly select the appropriate category for the right situation. Figure 4.9 shows some examples of nursing situations in which one particular category can be used. They can *only* be examples. It is acknowledged that the stated category would always be used *along with* others. The examples do, however, make concrete, the abstract: they show the practical application of the six category approach in everyday nursing life.

One last point needs to be made here; not *all* the categories will be

Prescriptive Interventions	1.	When delegating nursing duties.
	2.	Advising people prior to discharge
	3.	Enabling students to develop a conceptual framework.
Informative Interventions	1.	During the admission of new patients.
	2.	Reporting to other health professionals.
	3.	During teaching sessions.
Confronting Interventions	1.	When anti-social behaviour occurs.
	2.	When incorrect nursing procedures are used.
	3.	During multi-disciplinary meetings.
Cathartic Interventions	1.	Whilst counselling relatives.
	2.	Whilst caring for the spiritually distressed
	3.	Whilst caring for the dying.
Catalytic Interventions	1.	During clinical teaching sessions.
	2.	Whilst talking to patients whilst compiling care plans.
	3.	Whilst counselling the distressed or uncertain person.
Supportive Interventions	1.	During all nursing situations.
	2.	During all teaching situations.
	3.	Throughout all human interactions.

Fig. 4.9   *Examples of nursing situations in which skills of a particular category may be used*

used in *every* social or therapeutic encounter. As we have noted all along, the point is to be able to skilfully choose the right approach at the right time.

Also, it may not be for nothing that the nurses in our study felt themselves to be most skilled in being supportive. Everyone needs support and encouragement. Everyone needs to be affirmed. Or as Martin Buber put it:

> 'Man wishes to be confirmed by man ... secretly and
> bashfully he watches for a Yes which allows him to be
> and which can only come from one human person to
> another.' (Buber, 1965).

Exercises in the six categories

The following exercises allow for three phases of personal development:

1. The ability to discriminate between the categories

2. Ability to use each category skilfully
3. Applications of the categories to the counselling situation and to the wider nursing context.

Exercise 11

Aim of the exercise: To enhance discrimination between the six categories of therapeutic intervention.
Group size: Any number from 6 to 20.
Time required: Between 40 minutes and 1 hour.
Materials and/or environment required: A large, comfortable room and a circle of straight-backed chairs.

Process

1. The facilitator describes the six categories as outlined above.
2. Group members in turn state a category title and then offer an example of an intervention in that category, e.g. 'Catalytic intervention: "Can you tell me more about what happened?"'.
3. The group decide whether or not the example offered was a true example of an intervention in the stated category.
4. When all group members have offered a category title and an example, a discussion is developed about the use of the analysis.

Evaluation

The facilitator may want to ask:

● What sorts of interventions do you find yourself commonly using?
● What particular interventions do you feel least happy using?

Exercise 12

Aim of the Exercise: To enhance discrimination between the six categories.
Group Size: Any Number from 6 to 20.
Time Required: Between 40 minutes and 1 hour.
Materials and/or Environment Required: A large, comfortable room and a circle of straight-backed chairs.

Process

1. Each group member in turn states, in the first person, something that he or she may say in a counselling situation. They follow the expression by 'tagging' it with a category label, as per the six categories, e.g. 'It is not possible for you to see the doctor today—informative intervention'.
3. When all group members have offered an expression and a 'tag', a discussion is developed about the use of the analysis.

Evaluation

The facilitator may ask the group:

- How accurate do you feel you are in identifying interventions?
- Were most of the interventions covered in that exercise?

Exercise 13

Aim of the exercise: To enhance discrimination between the six categories.
Group size: Any number from 6 to 20
Time required: About 1 hour
Materials and/or environment required: A large, comfortable room and a circle of straight-backed chairs. Notebooks and pens. A white or blackboard.

Process

1. The facilitator reads out each of the following expressions (or writes them on a white or blackboard).
2. Group members are invited to jot down which category each expression fits into.
3. Afterwards, the group discuss their findings.

The expressions are:

(a) 'What happened when you talked to your wife last night?'
(b) 'How are you feeling at the moment?'
(c) 'I am interested in what you have to say.'

(d) 'The tablets are likely to help the pain.'
(e) 'I suggest you talk to your daughter about this.'
(f) 'I would appreciate it if you stopped doing that'
(g) 'You feel angry at the moment?'
(h) 'I'm very fond of you'.
(i) 'It's O.K. to cry.'
(j) 'You could enrol on a course at night school.'
(k) 'You are laughing and you say you are angry ...'
(l) 'Who do I remind you of?'

Evaluation

The facilitator may want to ask:

● What are the problems associated with deciding on a particular category?
● Are there 'good' and 'bad' interventions?

Notes

Some group members are likely to want to know what the 'right' answers are. This can lead to a fruitful debate about personal perceptions and individual choices about what constitutes examples of each category.

Exercise 14

Aim of the exercise: To enhance discrimination between the six categories.
Group size: Any number from 6 to 20.
Time required: About 1 hour.
Materials and/or environment required: A large, comfortable room and a circle of straight-backed chairs. A pack of twenty four cards: four marked prescriptive, four marked informative and so on through the categories. The pack should be shuffled.

Process

1. The facilitator passes the pack of cards, face down, to the first group member.

2. The first member picks the first downturned card from the top of the pack and shows it to the group.
3. The group member then offers an example of an intervention from that category.
4. The group decides whether or not the intervention that was offered *was* a true example.
5. When the group is satisfied, the card is placed on the bottom of the pack and the pack is passed to the next group member.
6. Stages 2–5, above, are repeated.
7. When all members have completed the round, the facilitator leads a discussion on the outcome.

Exercise 15

Aim of the exercise: To identify individuals' and groups' strengths and deficiencies in the six categories.
Group size: Any number from 6 to 20.
Time Required: About 20–30 minutes.
Materials and/or environment required: A large, comfortable room and a circle of straight-backed chairs. A handout, laid out as shown in Fig 4.10 is required for each group member. A flipchart, chalkboard or whiteboard is required, on which is drawn the grid illustrated in Fig 4.11.

Process

1. The facilitator gives each member a handout laid out as shown in Fig 4.10.
2. Each group member ticks the two categories that he feels he currently uses most skilfully and puts crosses against the two that he feels he uses least skilfully.
3. When the handouts have been completed, the facilitator collates the results of the assessment on to the grid shown in Fig 4.11.
4. When the group reconvenes, a discussion is held on the outcomes.

Six category intervention analysis skills assessment
Please place a tick beside the *two* categories that you feel you currently use *most* skillfully, in any context. Place a cross beside the *two* categories that you feel you use *least* skillfully in any context.

	Most skilled	Least skilled
1. Prescriptive		
2. Informative		
3. Confronting		
4. Cathartic		
5. Catalytic		
6. Supportive		

Fig. 4.10   *Six category intervention analysis skills assessment form*

Evaluation

The facilitator may want to ask:

● How easy/difficult was this exercise to do?
● Does the ease with which you can use certain interventions depend on the *context*?
● Were you surprised by the outcome of this activity?

Notes

This is a very useful exercise to use at the beginning of a counselling skills workshop, once group members have grasped the essentials of the six category approach. Out of the collated results

	✓	✗
1. Prescriptive		
2. Informative		
3. Confronting.		
4. Cathartic.		
5. Catalytic.		
6. Supportive.		

Fig. 4.II *Six category intervention analysis skills assessment grid*

can be decided a format for concentrating on the development of particular categories that are identified as areas of weakness. Thus the activity becomes an aspect of the negotiated curriculum. It was this activity that gave us the idea to do the research into nurses' perceptions of their own interpersonal skills (Burnard and Morrison 1988, Morrison and Burnard, 1989) although different types of ranking and rating scales were used.

Exercises to develop skills in specific categories

Prescriptive skills

Prescriptive interventions involve giving advice, being critical, making suggestions and generally attempting to direct the behaviour of the other person. It is important that prescriptive interventions are made in the true interest of the other person. They should not degenerate into 'putting people's lives right' or into foisting your own set of values onto someone else. Nor should they patronize or oppress.

As a general rule, prescriptive interventions are probably best used to help with concrete life-problems. In other words, it is possible to give advice about, say, moving house or coping with diabetes; it is not so easy to give advice about how another person should live her life.

Exercise 16

Aim of the exercise: To explore the use of prescriptive interventions.
Group Size: Any number from 6 to 20.
Time required: About 1½ hours.
Materials and/or environment required: A large, comfortable room and a circle of straight-backed chairs. A flip chart pad, chalkboard or whiteboard.

Process

1. The facilitator displays the following list of situations.
2. Group members are invited to suggest whether or not they feel that a prescriptive approach would be suitable in helping with those situations.
3. After all of the items have been worked through, the facilitator leads a discussion on the problems of being prescriptive.

The situations are:

(a) A young patient asks you about how to cope with his colostomy.
(b) A student nurse wants to know how to cope with the fact that her boyfriend has left her.
(c) A staff nurse asks you what her next career move should be.
(d) A patient in a psychiatric unit asks you why he has been prescribed Orphenadrine and whether or not he should continue to take it.
(e) An elderly person asks you what she can do about the fact that she has lost her religious beliefs.
(f) A young girl asks you for your views on abortion.

Evaluation

The facilitator may want to ask the following questions:

● Can you identify when prescriptive interventions may be appropriate?
● What makes a 'good' prescriptive intervention?

Notes

Giving another person advice is a notoriously difficult thing to do. It is sometimes helpful if the phrase 'Can I make a suggestion ...?' precedes the advice. In this way (at least, in theory!), the other person can choose to listen to or avoid the advice.

Exercise 17

Aim of the exercise: To develop the use of prescriptive interventions.
Group size: Any number from 6 to 20.
Time required: Between 1 and 2 hours.
Materials and/or environment required: A large, comfortable room and a circle of straight-backed chairs.

Process

1. The facilitator invites the group to sit in silence for two minutes and to recall an incident from their lives in which they were given advice.
2. The group is then asked to divide into pairs.
3. Each pair nominates one of them as 'A' and the other as 'B'.
4. 'A' describes the incident to 'B' and 'B' listens without responding in any way.
5. After five minutes the facilitator asks 'A' to reflect upon the following questions:
   (a) How well was the advice given?
   (b) Was the advice appropriate?
   (c) How would *you* have delivered such advice?
   (d) Did you *take* the advice?
6. 'A' then ponders on these questions, aloud, in the presence of 'B'.

7. After five minutes, the facilitator asks the pair to exchange roles.
8. 'B' then relates his incident to 'A' and ponders on the above questions.
9. When the cycle has been completed, the facilitator invites the group to reconvene.
10. The group identifies the factors which contributes to the legitimate use of prescriptive interventions.

Evaluation

Questions similar to those outline for the previous exercise can be used here.

Notes

The philosopher, John-Paul Sartre maintained that we tend to ask advice from those people whose advice we could anticipate (Sartre 1973). In the end, we have to decide for ourselves.

Exercise 18

Aim of the exercise: To identify valid prescriptive interventions.
Group size: Any number from 6 to 20.
Time required: About 1 hour.
Materials and/or environment required: A large, comfortable room and a circle of straight-backed chairs.

Process

1. The facilitator invites each group member to offer an example of a prescriptive interventions, stated supportively and therapeutically.
2. After each intervention, the group decides:
   (a) Was the intervention an example of a prescriptive intervention?

(b) Was the manner in which the intervention was offered appropriate?

3. When all group members have offered an intervention, the facilitator convenes a discussion on the therapeutic use of prescriptive interventions.

Notes

This type of exercise is easily modified for *any* of the six categories and is useful for helping to 'cement' the concept of a particular intervention in people's minds.

Informative Skills

Informative interventions involve instructing, informing and generally imparting information to the other person. In counselling (and probably in most other situations), informative interventions are probably restricted to factual information and, as with prescriptive interventions, should not be about 'putting people's lives right'.

There has been great emphasis placed on information giving in nursing, in recent years (Hayward, 1975; Boore, 1978; Devine & Cook, 1983; Engstrom, 1984). It may be that nurses expect that an important part of their role is giving information to other people. This seems quite reasonable when such information is concerned with things like medicine, surgery and other 'factual' situations. It is of less certain value in areas where people are suffering from emotional and personal problems. Whatever the rights and wrongs of giving information, it is undeniable that information when it is given needs to be given clearly, unambiguously and supportively.

Exercise 19

Aim of the exercise: To develop the use of informative interventions.

Group size: Any Number from 6 to 20.

Time required: About 1 to 2 hours.

Materials and/or environment required: A large, comfortable room and a circle of straight-backed chairs. Flipchart sheets. Large felt-tipped pens.

Process

1. The facilitator divides the group into small sub-groups of 3–4 people.
2. Each person is asked to recall, silently, two people from their lives:

   (a) one who gave information badly;
   (b) one who gave information skilfully.

Examples may be drawn from parents, teachers, lecturers, friends and so forth.

3. In the small groups, group members identify on a flip chart sheet two lists of items:

   (a) the specific behaviours and qualities of the people who gave information badly;
   (b) the specific behaviours and qualities of the people who gave information skilfully.

4. After fifteen minutes, the group is invited to reconvene and share their findings.
5. The facilitator helps to draw out the necessary behaviours and qualities of the person who gives information skilfully and therapeutically.

Evaluation

The facilitator may want to ask the following questions:

- How effective are *you* at giving information?
- What are the most difficult things about giving information?
- What *sort* of information is difficult to give?

Notes

It is important that all group members are encouraged to practice their listening skills whilst doing these pairs exercises. A useful reminder is to every so often invite the pairs to 'freeze' at the end of an exercise and to notice the position that they and their partner is sitting in. This position can then be compared and contrasted with the SOLER behaviours described above.

Confronting skills

Confronting interventions involve being challenging or giving direct feedback to the other person about their behaviour, attitude and so forth. A confronting intervention challenges the restrictive attitudes, beliefs and behaviours of the other person. Examples of issues on which people may be confronted are identified in Fig 4.12.

Confronting interventions should always be offered supportively and they should never degenerate into an attack on the other person:

> Creative confrontation is a struggle between persons
> who are engaged in a dispute or controversy and who
> remain together, face to face, until acceptance,
> respect for differences, and love emerge; even though
> the persons may be at odds with the issue, they are no
> longer at odds with each other. (Moustakas, 1984).

Because the prospect of confronting another person often causes anxiety (for we risk being rebuffed, disagreed with or challenged ourselves), the temptation is either to:

(a) become aggressive and turn the confrontation into an attack. This is what Heron (1989a) calls the 'sledgehammer' approach;

or

(b) 'Pussyfoot', or timidly approach the topic without being clear what the confrontation is really about. The pussyfooter goes all round the houses in a usually vain attempt to avoid saying what he or she really mean.

- Direct feedback on behaviour, use of language, attitudes etc
- Direct feedback on the effects of the other person's behaviour on self and others
- Challenging illogicalities and inconsistencies
- Challenging incongruities between what is said and the 'body language' that accompanies it
- Challenging unaware, unconscious behaviour
- Drawing attention to contractful issues
- Drawing attention to rules or codes of conduct.

Fig. 4.12 *Examples of issues for confrontation*

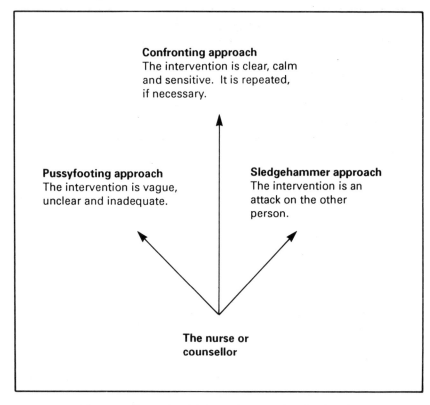

Confronting approach
The intervention is clear, calm
and sensitive. It is repeated,
if necessary.

Pussyfooting approach
The intervention is vague,
unclear and inadequate.

Sledgehammer approach
The intervention is an
attack on the other
person.

**The nurse or
counsellor**

Fig. 4.13   *Range of possible interventions either side of confrontation*

Fig 4.13 shows a possible range of interventions from the sledge-hammer through to the pussyfoot and identifies confrontation as the centre point. Using confrontation well takes practice. The nature of the nursing profession is such that nurse often feel unable to assert themselves and confront 'cleanly'. As a result, the outcome is often that they either attack or avoid. Our research suggested that confrontation is the skill that some nurse find the most difficult of all the six in this analysis (Burnard and Morrison, 1988, Morrison and Burnard, 1989). Assertiveness training can help here (Bond, 1986) and courses in assertion training are frequently offered by colleges and extra-mural departments of universities. They can be a useful way of developing confronting skills and of furthering self-awareness.

Exercise 20

Aim of the exercise: To practice the use of confronting interventions
Group size: Any number from 6 to 20
Time required: About 2 hours
Materials and/or environment required: A large, comfortable room and a circle of straight-backed chairs.

Process

1. The facilitator explains that this exercise involves role-play and invites the group to break up into sub-groups and decide upon:
   (a) two 'characters'
   (b) one or two process observers
2. When the sub groups have assembled the following instructions are given:
   (a) One character is a student nurse
   (b) One character is a charge nurse
   (c) The student nurse has been reported to the charge nurse regarding one of the following issues:
      (i) she is persistently late
      (ii) she has made sexual advances towards another member of staff.
         OR
      (iii) she has been abusive towards a number of patients.
   (d) The charge nurse's task is to meet the student and to confront her on the issue. The charge nurse should be clear, calm and supportive and avoid either the pussyfooting or the sledgehammer approaches.
   (e) The process observer's task is to observe the role-play unfolding and to rate the charge nurse on her ability to be skilfully confronting.
3. After the role-play has run for fifteen minutes, the facilitator invites each sub-group to evaluate their experience in the following manner:
   (a) The charge nurse self-evaluates her performance

(b) The student nurse evaluates the charge nurse's performance

(c) The process observers offer their observations to the charge nurse.

It is important that only the charge nurse's performance is under review. How ever effective the person was playing the student nurse, the aim is to concentrate on effective confrontation, not on the quality of the acting!

3. When the whole cycle of events has been completed, the facilitator reconvenes the larger group and invites feedback from the sub-groups.

4. Following the plenary session, the group collectively identify what behaviours and qualities make for successful confrontation.

Evaluation

The facilitator may want to ask:

● What are *you* like at confrontation?
● What are the specific problems involved in confronting another person?
● *Who* do you confront best?
● Who would you *least like* to confront?

Notes

As this is role-play, it is important that the people who have been role-playing are de-briefed after the exercise. This may be achieved by each actor disassociating from the role by describing to the group one of the following:

(a) A recent pleasant experience,
(b) Interests away form the group and away from work,
(c) Their job in real life.

This exercise can be adapted to suit the particular nursing group taking part. More difficult topics can be chosen for more senior staff. Groups may also be invited to choose their own topics for role play.

The technical details of trade union representation and the grievance procedure do not normally go unquestioned during this activity and can serve as useful material for discussion!

Cathartic Skills

Being human is a complicated business. It is complicated further by our emotional makeup. We experience joy and pain, laughter and disappointment. We also all have a tendency to bottle up emotion. Cathartic interventions are those that help the other person to explore their feelings and, as necessary, to express them, through laughter, anger, trembling or tears. We live in a culture where the free expression of feelings is not the norm. Given that they are often helping people who are likely to be emotional, it is important that nurses learn skills in helping in this domain.

Types of emotion

John Heron (1977) distinguishes between at least four types of emotion, that are frequently suppressed or bottled up; anger, fear, grief and embarrassment. He suggests a relationship between these feelings and certain overt expressions of them. Thus, anger may be expressed as loud sound, fear as trembling, grief through tears and embarrassment through laughter. He notes, also, a relationship between those feelings and certain basic human needs. Heron argues that we all have the need to understand and know what is happening to us. If that knowledge is not forthcoming, we may experience fear. We need to make choices in our lives and if that choice is restricted in certain ways, we may feel anger. Thirdly, we need to experience the expression of love and of being loved. If that love is not forthcoming or if it is taken way from us, we experience grief. To Heron's basic human needs may be added the need for self respect and dignity. If such dignity is denied us, we may feel self-conscious and embarrassed. Figure 4.14 illustrates some of the effects of bottling up emotion over a long period.

Coping with other people's emotions

Different people react in different ways to the bottling up of emotion in the same way. Some people, too, choose not to deal with life events emotionally. It would be odd to argue that there is a 'norm' where emotions are concerned. On the other hand, many people complain of being unable to cope with emotions and if the person being

- Physical discomfort and muscular pain; particularly muscular discomfort
- Difficulty in decision making
- Problems with self-image
- Difficulty in setting realistic goals
- The development of long term faulty beliefs
- The 'last straw' syndrome; lashing out at objects or at other people.

Fig. 4.14   *Some effects of bottling-up emotion*

counselled perceives there to be a problem in the emotional domain, then that perception may be expressed as a desire to explore his or her emotional status. It is important, however, that nurses do not force her particular set of beliefs about feelings and emotions on the other person, but waits to be asked to help. There should be no question that we force cathartic counselling on others under the belief we may have that emotional release is 'good for you'. Sometimes it is: sometimes it isn't.

Drawing on the literature on the subject, the following statements may be made about the handling of emotions:

- emotional release is usually self-limiting. If the person is allowed to cry or get angry, that emotion will be expressed and then gradually subside.
- there seems to be a link between the amount we can 'allow' another person to express emotion and the degree to which we can handle our own emotion. This is another reason why nurses need self-awareness. To help others explore their feelings we need, first, to explore our own.
- touch can often be helpful in the form of holding the person's hand or putting an arm round them. Care should be taken, however, that such actions are unambiguous: for some, touch always has sexual connotations. It is worth remembering, too, that not everyone likes or wants physical contact. It is important the nurses's support is not intrusive.
- once the person has had a emotional release they will need time to piece together the insights that they gain from such release. Often all that is needed is that the nurse sits quietly with the other person while he occasionally verbalizes what he is thinking. The post cathartic period can be a very important stage in the cathartic process.
- Certain counselling interventions can help in the exploration of feelings and in the promotion of emotional release. These are illustrated in Fig 4.15

Type of cathartic intervention	Example
1. Giving Permission	'It's all right with me if you cry ...'
2. Helping remove physical blocks.	'Try taking three deep breaths ... open your eyes really wide ...'
3. Picking up on sudden physical gestures.	'Try exaggerating that arm movement ... that facial expression ...'
4. Noting mismatches between verbal and non-verbal behaviours.	'You say you're upset and you're smiling.'
5. Inviting repetition of emotionally charged statements, offered by the client.	'Try saying "I'm angry", again ... and again ...'
6. Exploring fantasy.	'If you could do whatever you wanted, what would you do?'
7. Mobilization of body energy.	'Stand up and stretch ... shake yourself vigorously.'
8. Literal description of a place that the client has talked about.	'You talked about your old house ... describe one of the rooms to me ... in detail.'
9. Exploring hidden agendas.	'Who are you *really* saying that too?'
10. Role-playing relationships.	'If your mother was here now, what would you say to her? What has been left unsaid?'
11. Catching fleeting thoughts.	Noting fleeting eye movements and asking: 'What are you thinking? .... What's the thought?'

Fig. 4.15 *Examples of cathartic interventions*

There are a number of ways in which the nurse can develop skills in exploring and expressing emotions in themselves and in others. Co-counselling offers a simple and effective means of gaining cathartic competence (Bond, 1986) Gestalt therapy workshops also help in the process of handling feelings. Both methods are frequently taught in short courses run by colleges and extramural departments of universities.

The examples shown in Fig 4.15 are but a few of many methods of helping in the expression of emotion. All of them, used deftly and

skilfully can enable client to explore their emotions. All of them, too
are also useful 'alternative' counselling techniques for helping to
liberate new trains of thought, fresh solutions and different perspectives on distressing issues. It is suggested that their use be explored
gently and carefully in training workshops and that nurses become
skilled in using them *with each other* before they begin to use them in
the clinical situation. It is also recommended that facilitators who
work a lot in the cathartic domain should first receive training in
cathartic methods.

Exercise 21

Aim of the exercise: To explore emotional areas in group
members' experience.
Group size: Any number from 6 to 20.
Time required: Between 1 and 1½ hour.
Materials and/or environment required: A large, comfort-
able room and a circle of straight-backed chairs.

Process

1. The facilitator explains that the aim of the exercise is to
   explore emotion and that expression of emotion during the exercise is quite acceptable.
2. The facilitator invites the group to divide into pairs.
3. Each pair nominates one of them as 'A' and one as 'B'.
4. 'A' talks to 'B', uninterrupted on one of the following topics:
   (a) early childhood experiences
   (b) my relationship with my family
   (c) what I would tell you about myself if I knew you really well
   (d) What I worry about most of all
   (g) What makes me happy and unhappy.
5. 'B' gives 'A' attention only and does not interrupt.
6. After ten minutes, 'A' and 'B' exchange roles and work through
   the exercise again.
7. After all group members have completed the cycle, the group
   reconvenes and discusses the experience. There should, however, be no discussion of the content of the pairs' work. That

should remain confidential to the pairs concerned. Instead, the discussion should focus on what the *feelings* generated.

8. At the end of the allotted time, the facilitator invites each member of the group to describe something that he or she is looking forward to. This serves to 'lighten' the atmosphere and to end the session on a positive note.

Evaluation

The facilitator may like to ask:

- What sorts of *feelings* emerged?
- What did you *do* with those feelings?
- How do you normally cope with your own feelings?
- What do you do when other people express emotion?

Exercise 22

Aim of the exercise: To practice the use of cathartic interventions.
Group size: Any number from 6 to 20.
Time required: Between 1 and ½ hours.
Materials and/or environment required: A large, comfortable room and a circle of straight-backed chairs.

Process

1. The facilitator outlines a variety of cathartic interventions and demonstrates their use.
2. The group divided into pairs.
3. Each pair nominates one of them as 'A' and the other as 'B'.
4. 'A' talks to 'B' and 'B' uses a limited number of cathartic interventions from the list above. Only cathartic interventions are used. Suitable topics for the exercise are:
   (a) My feelings about my life so far
   (b) My feelings about my family
   (c) My relationships with close friends
   (d) My relationship with myself
5. After ten minutes, the pairs swop roles

6. When all group members have completed the cycle of events, the facilitator reconvenes the group and invites a discussion on the experiences of group members. Again, the content of what was talked about is not discussed. The focus of the discussion should be:
   (a)   the feelings of group members
   (b)   the ease or difficulty of using cathartic interventions.

Notes

It is sometimes helpful if a video taped can be prepared and shown to the group on the skilled use of cathartic interventions. Alternatively, the facilitator can demonstrate their use with a skilled person brought into the group for the purpose.

Catalytic Skills

> When you ask me how I feel, I'm the only one who
> can tell you! And I like that! (Primary school child
> quoted by Canfield and Wells 1976)

Catalytic interventions are those that involve drawing the person out through the use of open questions, reflection and empathy building. Examples of such interventions are illustrated in Fig 4.16.

Exercise 23

Aim of the Exercise: To discriminate between open and closed questions.
Group size: Any number from 6 to 20.
Time required: Between 40 minutes and 1 hour.
Materials and/or environment required: A large, comfortable room and a circle of straight-backed chairs. Handouts marked O.C.C.O.O.C.

Process

1. The facilitator demonstrates the difference between open and closed questions,
2. The group divides into pairs,

Open questions:
An open question is one that has potential for the client to develop. It does not require a 'yes' or a 'no' answer.
e.g. 'How do you feel about what's happening at home?'
Open questions tend to begin with: 'How', 'What', 'When' or 'Why'.

Reflection
Reflection is the technique of repeating or paraphrasing the last few words of the other person's utterance, e.g.
Client: 'I left home and found life very difficult. I couldn't settle and didn't know what I should do ...'
Nurse: 'You weren't sure what to do ....'
It is helpful if 'reflections' do not become 'questions', through the nurse's tone of voice and inflection. The 'reflection' should be a 'mirror' image of the last few words spoken by the other person.

Empathy building
Empathy building involves the nurse intuitively assessing the feeling of the other person and verbalizing that assessment, e.g.
'You sound very angry'
'That must have been very upsetting ...'

Fig. 4.16   *Examples of catalytic interventions*

3. Each pair nominates one of them as 'A' and one as 'B'.
4. 'A' then asks questions of 'B' in the order on the handouts (open, closed, closed, open, open, closed).
   Suitable topics for this exercise include:
   (a) The River Thames
   (b) Veteran cars
   (c) Steel tubes
   (d) Favourite pictures.
   These topics are useful because they elicit short answers and thus keep the exercise brisk. If emotive or interesting (!) topics are used, the exercise is likely to take a long time and the point of sticking to open and closed questions may be lost.
5. At the end of the first cycle of questions, the pairs exchange roles and the other person works through the list of questions.
6. When all group members have asked the series of questions and have been asked questions, the facilitator invokes a discussion on the process of asking questions.

Evaluation

The facilitator may like to ask:

- When would you use open questions in preference to closed questions?
- When would closed questions be appropriate?
- What sort of questions do you ask most frequently in the clinical situation?

Exercise 24

Aim of the exercise: To explore the use of 'why' questions.
Group size: Any number from 6 to 20.
Time required: Between 1 and 2 hours.
Materials and/or environment required: A large, comfortable room and a circle of straight-backed chairs.

Process

1. The facilitator invites the group to break into pairs.
2. Each of the pairs nominates one of them as 'A' and one as 'B'.
3. 'A' then talks to 'B' about his or her effectiveness as a counsellor.
4. As the conversation unfolds, 'B' asks a continuous series of 'why' questions of 'A'.

Thus the conversation may sound a bit like this:

A: 'I am fairly good at talking to relatives ... except when they start getting emotional ...'
B: 'Why do you find it difficult when they get emotional?'
A: 'Because it makes *me* emotional, I suppose.'
B: 'Why does it make you feel emotional?'
A: 'It reminds me of my own problems ...'
B: 'Why does it do that?
And so on.

5. The pair continue in this way for ten minutes and then exchange roles. 'A' asks 'why' questions of 'B'.
6. When the exercise has been completed, the group reforms and the facilitator leads a discussion on what happened.

A Case in Point: Four

Andrew had completed a training course in behavioural therapy and later became a tutor. When he joined the teaching team he found them to be using a wide range of experiential learning methods. He had various heated debates about the philosophy behind the methods and dismissed the 'relativism' and subjective nature of much of the theory. Open-minded, he sat in on a few of his colleagues teaching and learning sessions and soon came to appreciate that many of the methods exactly echoed training activities that he had taken part in during his behavioural therapy. He realized that much of the debate had been about conceptual rather than practical matters and had focussed on the use of particular words rather than on what people did in the classroom. He realized, too, that humanistic psychology and behavioural psychology shared a fairly large number of ideas but use different words to describe them.

Evaluation

It is useful to consider the following questions:

- How did it feel to be asked a series of 'why' questions?
- What are the good and bad points about 'why' questions?
- How can 'why' questions be used in counselling?
- When are they best avoided?

Notes

This activity was developed out of Hinckle's 'laddering' process; a research method used to explore belief and value systems. It is described in greater detail by Bannister and Fransella (1986). The activity also explores the problems associated with asking 'Why?' questions in counselling.

Exercise 25

Aim of the exercise: To experience being asked a wide range of questions.

Group size: Any number from 6 to 20.
Time required: Between 1 and 1½ hours.
Materials and/or environment required: A large, comfortable room and a circle of straight-backed chairs.

Process

1. The facilitator invites the group to divide into pairs.
2. Each pair nominates one of them as 'A' and one as 'B'.
3. 'A' asks 'B' questions on *any topic at all*, continuously.
4. 'B' *does not answer* any of the questions but merely experiences the feelings that go with being asked them.
5. After ten minutes, 'A' and 'B' exchange roles.
6. When all the group members have completed the cycle, the group facilitator invites the group to reconvene and to discuss the experience.

Evaluation

The facilitator may want to ask:

● What did it feel like *not* to answer questions?
● Did anyone break the rule?
● Did you answer the questions 'silently'?
● What is it like to be bombarded with questions?

Notes

This can be a powerful exercise for demonstrating how intrusive some forms of questioning can be. The facilitator may want to suggest that the group members ask some 'risky' questions—reminding them that at no time are *answers* required!

Exercise 26

Aim of the exercise: To develop the use of reflection.
Group size: Any number from 6 to 20.
Time required: Between 40 minutes and 1 hour.
Materials and/or environment required: A large, comfortable room and a circle of straight-backed chairs.

Process

1. The facilitator describes and demonstrates the technique of reflection.
2. The facilitator asks the group to divide into pairs.
3. Each pair is nominated 'A' and 'B'.
4. 'A' talks to 'B' and 'B' reflects appropriately. Reflection is the only intervention used. Any topic may be chosen for this activity.
5. After ten minutes, 'A' and 'B' exchange roles and repeat the process.
6. When all group members have worked through the cycle, the facilitator invites the group to reconvene and encourages discussion of the difficulties and value of reflection.

Evaluation

The facilitator may want to ask:

- When would you use reflection?
- When would you avoid it?

Notes

It is interesting to show a video tape of a television interview as an example of the effective use of reflection. Alternatively, the facilitator may ask a colleague to come into the room and demonstrate effective reflection with the facilitator.

Exercise 27

Aim of the exercise: To develop a range of catalytic interventions.
Group size: Any number from 6 to 20.
Time required: Between 1 and ½ hours.
Materials and/or environment required: A large, comfortable room and a circle of straight-backed chairs.

Process

1. The facilitator asks the group to divide into pairs.
2. Each pair nominates one of them as 'A' and one as 'B'.

3. 'A' talks to 'B' using only the following sorts of interventions:
   (a) open questions
   (b) reflections
   (c) empathy building statements

   Thus 'A' initiates the conversation with 'B'.

4. After ten minutes, the facilitator invites the pairs to exchange roles.

5. When all group members have completed the cycle, the facilitator encourages a discussion on their experiences.

Evaluation

The facilitator may want to ask:

- Which sorts of interventions were most difficult to use?
- Which were easiest to use?

Notes

A useful variation on this exercise is to invite the pairs to use the catalytic interventions as clumsily as possible. As we noted previously, 'doing it wrong' can often be a powerful training tool.

This exercise is the first one in which 'A' *initiates* a conversation. It is a useful activity for enabling nurses to consider how to start a conversation with a patient, relative or colleague.

Supportive Skills

Supportive interventions are those that involve approving, confirming or validating the other person's experience. The interventions should be genuine, appropriate and never patronising, paternal or maternal. Neither should they be used 'automatically' as positive reinforcement. It is notable that some nurse are compulsive carers and may *overuse* the supportive category. Overuse of support encourages dependence and disallows the other person from learning from their own experience through standing on their own feet.

Exercise 28

Aim of the exercise: To develop the use of supportive interventions.

Group size: Any number from 6 to 20.
Time required: Between 1 and 1½ hours.
Materials and/or environment required: A large, comfortable room and a circle of straight-backed chairs.

Process

1. each group member receives validation from each other member of the group. In order to facilitate this, the sentence:
   'The qualities I like most about you are ...'
   may be used. The validatory comments should be genuine and unqualified. Look out for statements that have a 'but' in them!
2. When each member of the group has received validation from every other member, the facilitator invites discussion on the experience.

Evaluation

The facilitator may want to ask:

● What did it feel like to be validated in this way?
● Where there any surprises?
● Did you enjoy the process?
● How effective are you at telling patients and other colleagues that you like them?

Exercise 29

Aim of the exercise: To explore self-validation.
Group size: Any number from 6 to 20.
Time required: About 1 hour.
Materials and/or environment required: A large, comfortable room and a circle of straight-backed chairs.

Process

1. Each member of the group, in turn, identifies three or four of their *own* positive characteristics or qualities, to the group.
2. When each person has spoken in this way, the facilitator leads a discussion on self-perception.

Evaluation

The facilitator may want to ask:

- What were other people's views of the qualities chosen by individuals?
- Does anyone want to *add* qualities to the lists that people offered?

Conclusion

When individual categories of interventions have been developed, the group may take longer periods in the pairs format attempting to use the whole range of categories. Alternatively, group exercises may be used such as the ones for discriminating between the categories as described at the beginning of this section.

Once the exercises have been experienced, a commitment must be made by each group member to practice the use of the interventions in the clinical situation. The exercises are of little value if the learning from them stays within the group or within the room. It is vital that the interventions become incorporated into the person's personal style. Once this is the case, the need to notice what interventions we are using becomes less necessary; the interventions have become the person. Sometimes the transitional phase between first learning to discriminate between the six categories and successfully incorporating them into self-presentation is experienced as a period of clumsiness and self-consciousness. Any new learning and any new skills development must cause changing in the sense of self and such a period normally passes into one of the development of a natural, spontaneous sense of self which is broadened and deepened by the wider choice that the analysis offers.

What has been argued and developed in this chapter is that the skilled nurse has self-awareness. Nurses can *choose* the interventions that are to be used and use them both skilfully and appropriately. Such skilled people have both listening and attending skills. They are skilled in making suggestions, giving information, challenging, drawing out, helping to release emotion and supporting. All of these skills need to be practised in an atmosphere of concern for, and appreciation of, the worth of the other person. The development of these human skills through personal experience will enhance and enrich the nurse's approach to patient care.

These are the skills and qualities of the one-to-one relationship. In the next chapter, the group process is examined and exercises in developing group skills are explored. Finally, in this chapter, a programme for using the attending, listening and counselling skills exercises is offered as a framework for planning a workshop or course.

(A) Programme for counselling skills training

1. Introductions:
   (a) The group facilitator introduces the aims of the workshop and outlines domestic arrangements: meal breaks and tea and coffee breaks.
   (b) the facilitator invites the group members to introduce themselves using the approach outlined in this book. Icebreakers can also be used as required.
   (c) the facilitator discusses the aims of the workshop and introduces the two principles:
      (i) the voluntary principle: that everyone is free to take part in activities or to sit out of them as they see fit,
      (ii) the proposal clause: that group members should take responsibility for suggesting that the group either spends more time on a certain section of the workshop or that things are speeded up.

2. Theory input
   (a) the facilitator offers a short theory input on the principles of counselling, including:
      (i) definitions of counselling
      (ii) qualities of an effective counselling
      (iii) how counselling fits into nursing practice
   (b) the facilitator makes a distinction between two aspects of counselling skills:
      (i) attending and listening
      (ii) counselling interventions

3. Experiential Learning Activities
   (a) the group then concentrates on attending and listening skills and work through a series of exercises (e.g. exercises No. 1–10 from this book).
   (b) after a plenary session to discuss all aspects of attending and listening, the facilitator moves the group on to counselling interventions.
   (c) the concept of Six Category Intervention Analysis is introduced and discussed and group members assess their own

skills in terms of the six through using the assessment sheet outlined on page 122.

(d) out of that assessment, a group profile is drawn up using the grid on page 123.

(e) the group then concentrate on the three categories that are generally perceived as those requiring most attention.

(f) the group work through a series of exercises to develop skills in the six categories (e.g. a selection from exercises 11–29 from this book).

(g) group members are encouraged to work in pairs for longer periods (between ½ and 1 hour as 'A' or 'B') to reinforce the skills learned.

Evaluation and application

(a) a final plenary session is held to discuss the application of the new skills to the clinical or community setting.

(b) the facilitator leads a evaluation session and closes the workshop.

This format can be adapted for use as a one or two day workshop, a week long workshop or as a series of study days.

5

Experiential Exercises for Human Skills—Group Skills

> ... an ability to be healing or therapeutic is far more common in human life than we might suppose. Often it needs only the permission granted by a freely flowing group experience to become evident (Rogers, 1972).

We all live and work in a variety of types of groups. If the counselling process as outlined and discussed in the previous chapter is comparable to any one-to-one encounter, similarly the group process mirrors any situation in nursing in which three or more people meet. In the nursing profession the individual joins many groups; the training and educational group in the school of nursing, the nursing team on the ward, a variety of meetings, case conferences and so forth. Figure 5.1

Ward reports/handovers
Case conferences
Ward policy meetings
Unit meetings
Educational groups
Therapy groups
Relaxation groups
Stress management workshops
Study days
Interdisciplinary meetings
Management meetings
Professional issues meetings
Union meetings
Planning meetings
Relatives meetings
Clinical teaching groups

Fig. 5.1   *Examples of nursing groups*

identifies some of the many groups that are used in the profession. In groups the individual may play many parts and the group often causes the individual to act differently to the way she would in a one-to-one meeting.

Various skills are required both to be a successful group member and to be a group leader or facilitator. Before such skills are discussed, it may be useful to have an overall map of the group process as a means of understanding the stages through which every group, of every sort, seems to pass.

A Map of the Group Process

Figure 5.2 offers such a map, based on the word of Tuckman (1965). He noted that every group passes through four stages in its development and life. He described these as the stages of (a) forming,

---

Stage one: the forming stage
- group members meet
- members hesitantly get to know each other
- trust and disclosure are low
- there is minimal achievement by the group

Stage two: the storming stage
- the group explores relationships between its members
- there is infighting and conflict between group members
- there are tensions between the needs of the individual and the needs of the group.

Stage three: the norming stage
- the group establishes rules for itself; both explicit and tacit
- arguments and disagreements are settled
- those who are likely to leave have usually left
- the group becomes cohesive

Stage four: the performing stage
- the group becomes mature and productive
- group members accept individual differences between themselves
- the group can work together
- the group has come of age
  BUT
- there is a danger of stagnation and of 'groupthink'

Fig. 5.2 *An overview of the group life cycle (after Tuckman, 1965).*

(b) storming, (c) norming and (d) performing. During stage one, the forming stage, group members meet each other for the first time and attempt to discover what behaviour is and is not required of them. This is a time for testing the water, of discovering other people and for discovering one's role in the group. In many ways, the new member of the group is 'on her best behaviour': the real person has yet to emerge.

In the storming stage, group members begin to thaw out a little. As a result they characteristically become hostile with one another as they battle to assert themselves and to stamp their personalities on the group. This is the stage of conflict between 'my' needs and wants and those of the group. Often this is a painful period in which there are fights for leadership of the group and attempts at establishing a pecking order. Nurses in the early stages of their nursing education and training, for example, may notice the advent of the storming stage developing once the introductory period in the school or college has been worked through or towards the middle or end of their first year. In this stage, friendships and loyalties are tested and it may be a time when certain individuals either opt out of the group and leave the education and training course or feel pressurized to leave by the group.

Out of the storming stage develops the 'norming' stage, when the group comes to terms with itself and the individuals in it resolve their conflicts to some degree—both personal and interpersonal. In order for the group to function harmoniously, rules, both written and unwritten, are established in the group's resolve to become more cohesive. Members typically get to know one another better and are a more trusting, intimate atmosphere develops. Nurse education and training courses when they reach this stage are often perceived as having established themselves by their tutors or lecturers and fellow nurses. The group feels as though it has arrived!

The danger, here, is that such groups will become *too* settled and too complacent. There is also a problem when groups are too readily socialized into the norms of the institution. In this case, they tend to be readily accepting of what they see and lose a certain critical faculty. It is important that all nurses maintain the ability to think critically and are able to challenge the prevailing practices in the clinical areas in which they work. In most large institutions there develops what has been called an 'organizational culture' (Sathe, 1983). That is to say that institutions, as large groups themselves, develop their own norms and seek to initiate newcomers into those norms in order for things to go along much as they have in the past. The new nursing group not only has to develop its own norms but may find itself in conflict or disagreement with the norms of the organisational culture.

The norming stage leads on to the most productive phase of group life; the performing stage. Here, the group has developed a mature collective identity and its members are able to work easily and usefully together. The danger arises, again, in this stage that the group can become complacent and that new growth is not encouraged. This can be seen in certain clinical environments were everyone has worked together for a considerable period and have come to know each other, their habits and behaviours, well. Such a group can become inward looking and reject both new ideas and new members. Consider, for example, some of the reaction that occurred when the nursing process was first introduced. A number of people in the profession suggested that: 'we don't need it; we function very well as we are, why change things?'. Students arriving in such groups often feel left out or feel that they are intruding. The group that arrives at the performing stage needs to keep itself alert to changes and suggestion from outside of itself. 'Groupthink,' the term that is sometimes used to describe the tendency for groups to work as if they were one, closed-minded individual, can occur if the group does not remain in touch and awake to other groups and to new ideas. It could be argued that many nursing groups and perhaps the profession itself has a tendency towards such closed thinking.

This then is a typical cycle through which most groups seem to pass. It may be viewed as a life-cycle of the group as is directly comparable to the life-cycle of the individual: it mimics childhood, adolescence, young adulthood and maturity. Thus the life cycle of life as experienced by the individual is played out in the larger arena of the group. Viewed in this light, the group experiences can be valuable for developing further individual awareness. The person who monitors his or her behaviour and responses in the group can gain insights into themselves through appreciating this correlation between the life cycle of the group and the life cycle of the individual. Nurses in the group may see themselves as 'reliving' stages of their own life when they join that group. The group is perhaps the most potent medium through which to develop self-awareness. In the group both self-disclosure and feedback from others are present— two vital ingredients for awareness.

If the metaphor of the life-cycle of the group is accepted, it will be understood that a group may well reach the point where it has fulfilled its function and the group is disbanded. The cycle has been completed. In nurse education and training this ending of the group life comes naturally at the end of a three or four year period because the life period for the group has been predetermined by the college, school or examining body. In other groups, however, such a time period may not be so clear cut and it is important that at periods through any 'performing' period, the group reviews its performance and function. There is little value in continuing the group's existence when the point of its existence has been exhausted. There is nothing worse that belonging to a 'dead' group.

Second to the issue of the group's stages comes the question of the processes that occur during the group's life. All that happens in a group may be divided into two aspects:

(a) content
(b) processes.

Content refers to all that is said and talked about in any given group. Processes are all those things that happen in a group: the dynamics of the group. Such processes occur in all groups of all types. They are more noticeable in small, intimate groups but also frequently occur in professional and work groups. They have been so frequently noted that they are easily described. Figure 5.3 identifies a variety of typical group processes that occur. Recognition of such processes is vital for anyone running groups and it is helpful if group members learn to recognise them. Once again, developing such awareness is part of the larger task of developing personal awareness. It is often useful if the group facilitator holds a discussion about group processes at one of the early meetings of that group. The facilitator may also like to invite group members to notice these processes as they occur, thus a sense of group reflexivity occurs. Time can then be put aside at regular intervals to discuss the perceived processes. In self-awareness groups, discussion of processes are just as important as the discussion of content. It is regrettable that traditional educational methods have mostly concentrated on the content of courses and study periods at the expense of exploring processes.

1. Pairing
Two group members talk to each other rather than to the group.

2. Projection
Group members blame 'the group', 'the organization' or 'nursing', for the way they are feeling, rather than owning the feeling.

3. Scapegoating
The group picks out one member to act as the person on whom to take out their hostile feelings.

4. Shutting down
A group member cuts his or herself off from the group and becomes isolated and often emotionally distraught.

5. Rescuing
A group member constantly serves as the person who defends other members of attack. Sometimes, the facilitator may *have* to rescue.

6. Flight
The group avoids serious issues by taking avoiding action; talking light-heartedly, intellectualizing or changing the topic.

Fig. 5.3 *Examples of group processes*

Group Processes

Typical group processes may thus be described. Pairing can be noted when two individuals, usually sitting next to each other, engage in a quiet and often hesitant conversation with each other. The conversation may occur as a series of 'asides', facial expression and, in the extreme form, in the passing of notes! Pairing is distracting for other group members and may occur as a result of disaffection with the group, insecurity on the part of one or both of the pair involved, boredom or as a means of testing group leadership. Another form of pairing can be seen when two group members form a fairly exclusive relationship and support each other in a determined manner whenever either of them makes a contribution to group affairs and particularly when either of them is under attack from any other group member.

Projection occurs when individuals identify the group as being responsible for their feelings. Individuals see a quality in the group which is, in fact, a quality of their own but of which they are unaware. Thus individuals may say 'this group is hostile and unfriendly', when it is plain to the rest of the group that such a description fits the individuals themselves herself. Such projection may arise out of insecurity in the group or out of the individual's own lack of awareness. The process of 'owning' projections and taking responsibility for oneself can be a particularly valuable piece of experiential learning in the group. On the other hand, you have to be careful. Not *everything* that a person says about a group is a projection. Sometimes they are merely describing what is obviously true about the group. So how do you distinguish between a projection and a description? No easy task! Some guidelines that may help here are these:

(a) a projection is usually only experienced by one person,
(b) the rest of the group usually disagrees with a projection,
(c) often individuals come to recognize their own projections—especially if they are on the lookout for them,
(d) descriptions are usually corroborated by other group members,
(e) descriptions do not usually have the 'emotional tone' that can accompany projections.

Scapegoating often occurs during the 'storming' stage of the group. The group looks for someone to blame for the way they are feeling and behaving and chooses a fairly quiet or vulnerable member on whom to vent their feelings. In this sense, scapegoating is a type of collective bullying. Alternatively, the group finds an outside scapegoat and blames 'the organization' or 'the profession' for the circumstances in which it finds itself. This is the 'group beef'. Usually this blaming of outside organizations or bodies is a means of the group avoiding responsibility for itself or a way of avoiding making decisions. Recognition of such scapegoating is part of the group leader's role and identification of it by the group itself can lead to a sense of growing cohesion and personal awareness. Again, though, a word of caution. Sometimes the organization or the profession *is* to blame! It is important to make the distinction.

When a group member becomes 'shut down' (Heron 1973B), they cut themselves off from the rest of the group, often feeling swamped by it and emotionally fragile. This may be caused by the group member suddenly identifying with a painful experience that is being described by someone else. It may be a response to the general emotional tone of the group or it may be a rejection of the ideas that are being put forward in the group discussion. The skilled group facilitator recognizes such shutting down and helps the individual either to express his a her feelings or to quietly rejoin the group. There will be occasions, too, when the group member favours a short break from the group. Shutting down often occurs when a group member begins to face important emotional issues that have been previously buried. Shut down individuals are in crisis. They cannot face their feelings and cannot verbalize how they feel. Working through such a phase must be handled tactfully and sensitively and individuals should never be rushed or told that expressing their pent up feelings would 'do them good'. Sometimes it would: sometimes it wouldn't. The point is that it is the *group member*'s place to decide whether or not now is a good time to work through the bottled up feelings.

People who 'rescue' may be a 'compulsive carers'. They may find it easier to defend others from attack than to let those people fend for themselves and learn from the experience. Often rescuing others is a means of avoiding dealing with personal problems: to be seen as the person who always comes to another's aid can serve as a smokescreen for covering unresolved conflicts. It may be that many nurses are compulsive carers. Often it is easier to care for others than it is to care for ourselves. This is fine as far as it goes but constantly caring and rescuing others is a recipe for burnout and emotional exhaustion.

Part of the process of developing self-awareness includes our standing back and enabling others to learn through experience rather than rushing in and helping to quickly. Often the temptation is to protect others from that which we cannot take ourselves. We feel that 'if I can't take it, she can't', forgetting that the other person is a *different* person and blurring the distinction between 'me' and 'you'. As we gain awareness and resilience, we can 'allow' others to live through their own life without being over-protected or denied the chance to develop their own coping skills. This applies to a wide range of nursing situations: the patient who learns to cope with their anxiety develops the ability to cope with it again; the person who is allowed to live through a certain amount of pain, develops the ability to deal with pain. If we constantly 'rescue' we constantly deny people the ability to develop autonomy.

There are, of course limits to this. The group facilitator has responsibilities towards the members of his or her group and some judgments have to be made about the degree of rescuing that can be made. As a general rule, one may want to 'rescue' members who are being scapegoated in the early days of the group's development. As the group progresses, the facilitator can slowly rescue less and less and allow individuals to fend for themselves more and more.

The group process known as flight can be demonstrated in various ways. The group which avoids difficult issues or decisions can be said to be taking flight. The individual group member who is constantly humorous and lighthearted may also be taking flight in humour. The member who always has a theoretical explanation for everything may often be taking flight from feelings. Yet another form of flight is keeping group discussion and meetings on a superficial level, thus deep and more disturbing issues are kept safely at a distance. Identifying and working through flight is a means of helping the group to grow. Self-disclosure occurs more readily when flight is avoided and group members are able to share each other's experiences on an adult-to-adult basis.

Again, this is not to say that all laughter is flight or that the group should always be deep and profound. It is merely to acknowledge that we all escape from facing ourselves: especially in the company of others.

In looking at group processes, it is worth noting that the energy level of any group will fluctuate from time to time just as an individual's energy level will have its peaks and troughs. Part of the development of group life involves living through the periods of low energy and taking advantage of the peaks. Again, the skilful leader and skilful group member will *notice* such fluctuations, take responsibility for them and make adjustments as necessary. When group energy does drop, one of the following courses of action, by the facilitator, may be appropriate:

(a) sit it out and see what happens
(b) suggest a change of activity
(c) draw the group's attention to the drop in energy
(d) take a short break.

Characteristics of all groups

Finally, small groups have things in common. Dorothy Stock Walker (1987) offers a useful list of the characteristics of groups. The list is as follows:

1. Groups develop particular moods and atmospheres
2. Shared themes can build up in groups
3. Groups evolve norms and belief systems
4. Groups vary in cohesiveness and in the permeability of their boundaries
5. Groups develop and change their character over a period of time
6. Persons occupy different positions in groups with respect to power, centrality and being liked and disliked,
7. Individuals in groups sometimes find one or two other persons who are especially important to them because they are similar in some respect to significant persons in the individual's life or to significant aspects of the self
8. Social comparison can take place in a group
9. A group is an environment in which persons can observe what others do and say and then observe what happens next
10. A group is an environment in which persons can receive feedback from others concerning their own behaviour or participation.

Arguably, these characteristics are true of most small groups, from clinical case conferences to learning groups and from therapy groups to discussion groups. Walker's list offers considerable material for discussion with both peers and students and may be a useful starting point for the teaching about groups and group dynamics.

The theoretical and practical issues involved in group work are numerous. The bibliography at the end of this book includes references to other sources that take these and other issues further. It is important that a theoretical understanding of the nature of groups is essential for anyone who wants to work with groups on a regular and serious basis. Practical experience of groups is vital but this aspect is far easier to manage. As we have noted, we are all involved in group work throughout our professional lives. It is up to us to notice and be aware of the changing patterns and varying natures of those groups. It is through such observations that we learn how other people live and interact together.

In order to highlight some of the aspects of group work, the following exercises explore:

(a) the group experience from the point of view of being a member,
(b) group facilitation.

These exercises may be followed through systematically or specific ones may be chosen to highlight or experience a particular aspect of group work. It is often useful if these exercises are preceded by one or two 'icebreaker' exercises in order to help the group to relax and settle into the atmosphere of the session.

Exercises in group membership

In the following exercises, a clear aim is offered for each. This group may be told of this objective before carrying out the exercise or the group may carry out the exercise and make what they will of it. As we noted earlier, behavioural objectives are not particularly helpful in the experiential learning field; the whole focus of the enterprise is on the individual's subjective experience. Herein lies a conundrum. On the one hand, the facilitator clearly has something in mind when suggesting an activity. On the other, the facilitator is keen that group members learn what *they* need to learn from it. Sometimes to disclose an aim is to pre-empt the group's own learning from experience. Instead, when the aim is disclosed, the group helps to ensure that a self-fulfilling prophesy occurs: the group works towards achieving that aim. There is no easy answer to this. Probably a compromise is best. When it seems necessary to offer a rationale for a particular activity, disclose the aim. When the need is not so great, suggest the activity but not the aim.

Exercises similar to and variants of the following exercises may be found in a variety of sources. (See, for example, Arnold and Boggs, 1989; Kagan, Evans and Kay, 1986; Heron, 1973, 1989a; Canfield and Wells, 1976; Stevens, 1971; Burnard 1989b).

As was the case with the exercises in the previous chapter, it is important that participation in the group exercises is voluntary. If any member asks not to take part, such a request should be honoured without question. The member who chooses not to take part in this way may usefully serve as a process observer and offer feedback to the group once the exercise has been completed. It is notable that some people find group activities difficult and whilst they are quite happy to take part in pairs activities such as those described in the last chapter, they are less happy talking in front of the whole group.

Exercise 30

Aim of the exercise: To explore the relationships and perceptions of group members.
Group size: Any number from 6 to 20.
Time required: About 40 minutes.
Materials and/or environment required: A large, comfortable room and a circle of straight-backed chairs.

Process

1. The facilitator explains the exercise as follows
   Each group member arranges the rest of the group in order to form a family (e.g. 'David is my father, Sue my sister, Sian my cousin ...' and so on.)
2. When each group member has developed a family in this way, the facilitator develops a discussion about the activity.

Evaluation

The facilitator may want to ask:

- What did you feel about being part of someone else's 'family'?
- What did you think about the positions you were given?
- What does all this say about our relationships with each other?

Notes

A variation on this activity is for one 'family' to stay intact and to 'stay in role'. Relationships between 'family' members is then explored.

Exercise 31

Aim of the exercise: To develop group relationships and to highlight the occurrence of group processes.
Group size: Any number from 6 to 20.
Time required: Between 1 and 2 hours.

Materials and/or environment required: A large, comfortable room and a circle of straight-backed chairs.

Process

1. Group facilitator invite the group to discuss one of the following topics:

   (a) the caring relationship in nursing
   (b) the qualities of friendship
   (c) our relationships with each other

2. The group is asked to observe the following ground rules (which may be displayed on a large sheet of paper or given to the group in the form of a handout.)

   - Speak in the 'first person' (use 'I' rather than 'you', 'we' or 'people'. Thus, 'I am angry at the moment' rather than 'You always get angry when people treat you like that, don't you?')
   - Speak directly to other people, rather than *about* them. (Thus: 'I don't agree with you' in preference to 'I don't agree with what Gary says.')
   - Make statements rather than asking questions. (e.g 'I'm enjoying this', rather than 'Is everyone enjoying doing this?')
   - Avoid theorizing and explaining other people's behaviour (e.g. Avoid making statements such as: 'I think what James is really trying to say is ...' or 'What Ali really thinks is ...').

3. Facilitator indicate to the group *every* time a rule is broken and invite the person to rephrase their statement.

4. After one hour has elapsed, the rules are dropped and facilitator convene a discussion on the effects of using the rules.

Evaluation

The facilitator may want to ask:

- What was the experience like?
- Why did no one break the rules?
- What was it like when you did?

Notes

This set of rules is a useful one for enhancing clear communication and may be used as a set of 'ground rules' for a workshop or study day. Also, the group may be encouraged to monitor the ground rules themselves. It is always interesting when someone intentionally flouts all of them!

Exercise 32

Aim of the exercise: To encourage attention to the group and listening between members of the group.
Group size: Any number from 6 to 20.
Time required: Between 1 and 2 hours.
Materials and/or environment required: A large, comfortable room and a circle of straight-backed chairs.

Process

1. The group facilitator invites the group to discuss one of the following topics:
   (a) The problems of becoming self-aware
   (b) How I stop myself from becoming self-aware
   (c) Any other topic
2. The facilitator explains that after one member has spoken, any other member who wishes to speak must first *summarize* what the previous speaker has said. They may then make their own contribution.
3. This activity is carried on for about 1 hour and the group then reconvenes. The facilitator invokes a discussion on the exercise, without the summarizing rule.

Evaluation

The facilitator may want to ask:

● What problems did you have with this exercise?
● How well do you *normally* listen to other people in groups?

Notes

This exercise can also be used as a listening exercise in pairs. In this case, one person in the pair must always summarize what the other had said before making her own contribution. A similar approach was originally used by Carl Rogers as a method for developing client-centred counselling skills (Kirschenbaum, 1979).

Exercise 33

Aim of the exercise: To explore group processes without non-verbal cues.
Group size: Any number from 6 to 20.
Time Required: About 40 minutes.
Materials and/or environment required: A large, comfortable room and a circle of straight-backed chairs.

Process

1. The facilitator invites the group to turn their chairs around so that they all sit facing outwards, in a closed circle.
2. The facilitator then initiates a discussion on the topic of 'the importance of verbal and non-verbal communication'.
3. After 20 minutes, the group is asked to turn their chairs back round and to share their experiences.

Evaluation

The facilitator may want to ask:

● What did it feel like *not being able to see* the other members of the group?
● What are the advantages of not being able to see non-verbal behaviour?

Notes

This activity can be carried out in pairs to explore effective ways of communicating on the telephone. In this version, each pair sits back to back and holds a 'telephone conversation'. It may be used to explore breaking bad news over the telephone.

Exercise 34

Aim of the exercise: To experiment with the concept of shared leadership.
Group Size: Any number from 6 to 20
Time Required: About 2 hours.
Materials and/or environment required: A large, comfortable room and a circle of straight-backed chairs. A small cushion.

Process

1. The group facilitator describes the process of this activity as follows:
   (a) Only the person holding the cushion may talk,
   (b) A person wishing to say something must indicate that they want the cushion but must not speak until they hold it.
2. The facilitator places the cushion in the centre of the circle and invites the group to discuss one of the following topics, whilst observing the rules of the exercise:
   (a) Nursing models
   (b) Nursing theory
   (c) Nursing research
   (d) The idea of a leaderless group
   (e) any other topic
3. After one hour, the facilitator suggests dropping the rules and invokes a discussion on the exercise.

Evaluation

The facilitator may want to ask:

● Would it be possible to have a leaderless group in any other circumstances?
● Why did no one hold on to the cushion?

Notes

An interesting variation on this activity is for the facilitator not to suggest a topic for the exercise but to allow the group discussion to evolve spontaneously. This version is only recommended where group members know each other fairly well.

Exercise 35

Aim of the exercise: To explore the effects of silence in the group.
Group size: Any number from 6 to 20.
Time required: About 40 minutes.
Materials and/or environment required: A large, comfortable room and a circle of straight-backed chairs.

Process

1. The group facilitator invites the group to remain completely silent for ten minutes.
2. The facilitator breaks the silence at the end of the ten minute period and invokes a discussion on the feelings and experiences of the group during the silent period.

Evaluation

The facilitator may want to ask:

● How can silence in a group be dealt with?
● How do *you* normally cope with silences?

Notes

This activity is best carried out with a group of people that know each other fairly well.

Exercise 36

Aim of the exercise: To explore group feelings in a symbolic format
Group Size: Any number from 6 to 20
Time Required: Between 1 and ½ hours.
Materials and/or environment required: A large, comfortable room and a circle of straight-backed chairs. Large sheets of white paper. Paints, pastels, or coloured pencils for each person.

Process

1. The group facilitator asks each group member to draw an abstract or figurative picture of the group in any style that the person chooses. The facilitator emphasizes that no particular artistic experience is required.
2. On completion of the pictures, each member presents their picture to the group.
3. The facilitator then invites discussion on the significance of the pictures and invites comments on any similarities and differences between the various pictures.

Evaluation

The facilitator may want to ask:

● What do these symbols *mean*? (It is important that people are allowed to interpret *their own* pictures and that the facilitator does not rush to do this for them.)

Notes

The pictures may be displayed on the wall as a backdrop to a workshop or study day. It is also interesting to repeat this exercise with the same group at a later date and to compare the pictures from each occasion.

Exercise 37

Aim of the exercise: To explore self-disclosure and risk-taking.
Group size: Any Number from 6 to 20
Time Required: Between 40 minutes and 1 hour.
Materials and/or environment required: A large, comfortable room and a circle of straight-backed chairs.

Process

1. The group facilitator invites each group member in turn to complete some of the following sentences. A 'round' of the group is completed before moving on to the next item.

(a) I am feeling ...
(b) What I am not saying at the moment is ...
(c) I could shock the group if I ....
(d) What I like most about this group is ...
(e) What I like least about this group is ...
(f) The topic that I find most difficult to discuss is ...
(g) I would be happier if this group ...
(h) If I could be anywhere else at the moment I would choose to be ...
(g) If I had to change places with a famous person, I would change places with ...

2. After the rounds have been completed the facilitator invites a free discussion on the exercise.

Evaluation

The facilitator may want to ask:

● What was it like waiting for your turn?
● Where any of the questions more statements more difficult than others?

Notes

The facilitator may invite the group to make up their own sentences for completion and also to facilitate the group whilst those sentences are being completed.

Exercise 38

Aim of the exercise: To explore similarities and differences between group members
Group size: Any number from 6 to 20.
Time required: Between 40 minutes and 1 hour.
Materials and/or environment required: A large, comfortable room and a circle of straight-backed chairs.

Process

1. The facilitator invites group members, in turn, to say:
   (a) who they feel is *most* like them in the group,
   (b) who is *most different* to them in the group.

2. The facilitator asks that group members do not give a reason for their choice at this stage.
3. When each member has had her turn, the facilitator invites a discussion on the perceptions of group members.

Evaluation

The facilitator may want to ask:

● What was it like being compared in this way?
● Where there any surprises?

Notes

It is important that the facilitator makes it clear that what is being asked is who is *most different* to the person concerned and not whom the other person *least likes*. This is a considerable shift in emphasis.

Exercise 39

Aim of the exercise; To explore group norms.
Group size: Any number from 6 to 20.
Time required: About 1 hour.
Materials and/or environment required: A large, comfortable room and a circle of straight-backed chairs. Large sheets of paper and pens.

Process

1. The facilitator hands out sheets of paper to each member of the group and asks them to draw three columns on the sheet.
2. Each person is invited to jot down ideas in the three columns as follows:
   (a) the norms that operate in this group,
   (b) the norms that operate in my home,
   (c) the norms that operate in this school or college of nursing.
3. After 20 minutes, the facilitator reconvenes the group and invites feedback on the activity. The sheets are displayed in the centre of the group.

Evaluation

The facilitator may want to ask:

- Are there great differences between norms in the three settings?
- If so, why is this the case?
- How did these norms come into being?
- Why?

Notes

Other norms can be explored in this way e.g.

(a) personal norms
(b) church norms
(c) ward norms
(d) secondary school norms
(e) norms in different classes in the school or college
(f) social norms.

Exercise 40

Aim of the exercise: To share positive, formative experiences in a group setting.
Group size: Any Number from 6 to 20.
Time required: Between 1 and ½ hours.
Materials and/or environment required: A large, comfortable room and a circle of straight-backed chairs.

Process

1. The facilitator invites the group to sit in silence for two minutes and to recall three positive, formative experiences from their childhood or up to the present time.
2. Group members then share those experiences with the group.
3. The group facilitator invites a discussion on formative experiences.

Evaluation

The facilitator may want to ask:

- *How* were these formative?

● Did you find that you thought of others but did not disclose them? (This should not be an invitation for further disclosure but can help people to become aware of what goes on 'just below the surface'.)

Notes

A challenging exercise for groups that know each other really well is for each member to also recall three *negative* experiences. if this format is used, it is recommended that the plan is as follows:

(a) the group members disclose and discuss *negative* experiences and then
(b) the group members disclose and discuss *positive* ones.

In this format the group closes on a positive note.

Exercise 41

Aim of the exercise: To explore members' perceptions of their position in the group.
Group size: Any number from 6 to 20.
Time Required: About 1 hour.
Materials and/or environment required: A large, comfortable room and a circle of straight-backed chairs.

Process

1. The group facilitator invites each member in turn to report to the group how they imagine the rest of the group sees them (e.g. 'I imagine that the group sees me as a fairly optimistic person with a lot to say and who sometimes talks too much ...').
2. After all members have had their turn, the group facilitator invites feedback to individual members, from the group.

Evaluation

The facilitator may want to ask:

● What were the difficulties with this activity?
● Did you enjoy it?

Exercise 42

Aim of the exercise: To explore self-disclosure and group decision making.
Group size: Any number from 6 to 20.
Time required: Between 40 minutes and 1 hour.
Materials and/or environment required: A large, comfortable room and a circle of straight-backed chairs. Sheets of lined paper for each person.

Process

1. The facilitator invites each group member to write down three topics that they would find very difficult to discuss. No further instructions are given.
2. When all group members have finished writing, the facilitator invites the group to decide democratically what is to be done with the sheets of paper. They may, for instance. decide to:
   (a) tear up the sheets
   (b) read out the items on the sheets
   (c) allow individuals to modify their sheets
   (d) pile up the sheets in the middle of the group and pick up someone else's sheet and then read that sheet aloud.
   (e) recall the sheets and rewrite them
   (f) disclose one item from the list.
4. After the process has been completed, the facilitator invokes a discussion on the exercise.

Evaluation

The facilitator may want to ask:

- Did *your* ideas about what should happen to the sheets coincide with what was decided?
- If not, how do you feel about that?
- What could you have done to change the decision?

Notes

A variation on this exercise is to invite people to jot down three things about themselves that they would find difficult to talk about.

An important point about this activity is that *any* individual who wishes to withdraw what they have written should reserve the right to do so at any time. This rule should override the decision made in the exercise.

Exercise 43

Aim of the exercise: To experience being asked questions by other group members and self-disclosing to the group.
Group size: Any number from 6 to 20.
Time required: Between 1 and 2 hours.
Materials and/or environment required: A large, comfortable room and a circle of straight-backed chairs.

Process

1. The facilitator explains that each group member, including themself, will spend three minutes being asked questions on any topic by the rest of the group. The individual in the 'hot seat' may choose to 'pass' on any question that they do not wish to answer.
2. One member volunteers to go first.
3. At the end of the three minutes, that person nominates another member of the group to take the 'hot seat' until everyone in the group has had a turn.
4. At any time, a group member may choose to 'pass' on the whole activity and not take her place in the 'hotseat'.
5. The facilitator should consider not passing on any question when it is her turn to take the hot 'seat.'
6. At the end of the process, the facilitator invites a discussion on the group's experience of the exercise.

Evaluation

The facilitator may want to ask:

- What sort of questions were asked mostly: open or closed?
- What motivated you to ask the questions that you did?
- What does all this tell you about the process of asking questions.

What the facilitator should not ask is why individuals 'passed' on certain questions.

Notes

This activity has numerous applications. It can, for instance be used with questions focused around a particular topic, as a revision aid. For example:

(a) nursing theory
(b) aspects of anatomy and physiology
(c) legal aspects of nursing
(d) ethical issues in nursing.

It can also be used in a shortened version as an icebreaker. Here, the time for questions is limited to 1½ minutes for each person.

Exercise 44

Aim of the exercise: To explore the use of touch in a group setting.
Group size: Any number from 6 to 20.
Time required: Between 40 minutes and 1 hour.
Materials and/or environment required: A large, comfortable room and a circle of straight-backed chairs.

Process

1. The facilitator invites the group to put on blindfolds or to close their eyes and keep them closed.
2. The facilitator then instructs the group to wander silently around the room.
3. As group members meet, they are invited to identify each other by touch alone. Once correct identification has been made, the person who has been identified can acknowledge who he or she is.
4. After all group members have be so identified, the facilitator encourages the group to reform and a discussion is held on the experience of the exercise.

A Case in Point: 5

Rebecca, who had been a nurse tutor for five years chose to attend a weekend workshop on experiential learning as a refresher course. The course was one that was open to anyone and was run as an encounter group. By the end of the first day, many people attending the workshop had cried and talked very openly about very personal matters. Rebecca was put off and decided not to go back for the second day. When she returned to the school, she became very dismissive of any experiential learning methods that were discussed or used.

A year later, a colleague pointed out that Rebecca was successfully using a whole range of listening exercises with groups of first year students. 'Yes', said Rebecca, 'but they are nothing to do with experiential learning'.

Evaluation

The facilitator may want to ask:

- What was it like to wander round blindfolded?
- Did you *hope* to identify certain people?
- Where there any surprises?

Notes

The facilitator should remain unblindfolded in order to ensure that group members to not hurt themselves through collisions with people or objects.

A variation on this activity is the traditional 'blind walk'. Here, group members pair off and one of each pair blindfolds themself. They are then led around by their partner to experience what it is like to be deprived of one sense. The pairs are encouraged to wander around outside the building, to attempt, carefully, the negotiation of stairs, to encourage the blindfolded person to touch objects, buildings, surfaces and so forth. A variant of *this* activity is for the blindfolded person only to be 'minded' by the other person. In other words, the pair wander round in silence and the blindfolded person does not hold the arm of the other person. The blindfolded person is apparently on her own. Both of these activities are powerful ones that are worthy of considerable discussion afterwards.

Exercise 45

Aim of the exercise: To identify relative roles and relationship of members of the group.
Group size: Any number from 6 to 20.
Time required: Between 30 minutes and 1 hour.
Materials and/or environment required: A large, comfortable room and a circle of straight-backed chairs.

Process

1. The facilitator invites the group to stand up and stand along an imaginary line, in the position that they feel the occupy in the group.
2. The facilitator may offer suggestions about the end points of the line: e.g.
   (a) quiet ... talkative
   (b) extrovert ... introvert
   (c) submissive ... dominant
   Alternatively, the facilitator may leave the group to decide on its own criteria.
3. When the line has been completed, the facilitator invites individual members to make changes to the order of the group as they see fit.
4. When the process has been completed, the facilitator invites the group to sit down and to discuss the implications of the line-up.

Evaluation

The facilitator may want to ask:

- Did you 'allow' yourself to be place in line or did you *decide*?
- Are their any other criteria for sorting people in this group?

Exercise 46

Aim of the exercise: To explore individual group members' perceptions of themselves.
Group size: Any number from 6 to 20

Time required: Between 40 minutes and 1 hour.
Materials and/or environment required: A large, comfortable room and a circle of straight-backed chairs.

Process

1. The facilitator invites group members to think of a household object *or* a piece of music *or* a book.
2. Each person in turn in then invited to describe themself as though they *were that object*, in the first person (e.g. 'armchair': 'I am soft and large and often get sat on by other people ...').
3. When each member of the group has had a turn, the group reconvenes and the facilitator leads a discussion on the exercise.

Evaluation

The facilitator may want to ask:

- Can you describe yourselves as objects that *other* people chose?
- What did you make of the descriptions?

Notes

As a variation on this activity, the facilitator may choose a category of item for each group member, thus:

(a) Imagine you are a piece of music ...what piece of music are you? Describe yourself as that.
(b) Imagine you are a piece of furniture ...what piece of furniture are you? Describe yourself.
(c) Imagine you are an animal ....what animal? Describe yourself.

Other categories that may be suggested are: a country, a book, a town, a river, a statue, a period in history, another person, a car, a building and so on.

Exercise 47

Aim of the Exercise: To explore spatial relationships between group members.

Group size: Any number from 6 to 20.
Time required: About 40 minutes.
Materials and/or environment required: A large, comfortable room and a circle of straight-backed chairs.

Process

1. The facilitator invites the group to wander round the room and to take time in finding the exact spot where they want to sit. Allow them to take plenty of time to do this.
2. From these positions, the group members are invited to share their thoughts on the significance of their positions.

Evaluation

The facilitator may want to ask:

● How did you choose *that* spot?

Notes

This activity may also be carried out with group members wearing blindfolds which are only taken off once everyone is seated. A discussion can then be held on the relative positions of everyone in the room.

Exercise 48

Aim of the Exercise: To share positive feelings for individual members and to enhance group cohesiveness.
Group size: Any number from 6 to 20.
Time required: Between 1 and ½ hours.
Materials and/or environment required: A large, comfortable room and a circle of straight-backed chairs.

Process

1. The facilitator invites each group member to listen to a 'round' of validating comments from each other group member. If

required, the incomplete sentence: 'The things I like most about you are ... may be used.

2. The group member being validated in this way receives the 'round without comment.'

3. When all the group members have taken part, the facilitator invokes a discussion on the exercise.

Evaluation

The facilitator may want to ask:

- Did you all *agree* with the comments that were made about you?
- What was it like to receive feedback of this sort?
- How skilled are you in telling people that you like them?

Notes

If group members know each other very well, a challenging exercise can be to invite *negative* feedback in the same format as above. The facilitator should ask that such feedback be given tactfully and supportively. This version should be used with care and only with the complete agreement of each member of the group. As with all the activities, individual members may reserve the right to opt out at any time during the activity.

Exercise 49

Aim of the exercise: To experience self and peer assessment in a group.

Group size: Any number from 6 to 20

Time required: Between 1 and 2 hours.

Materials and/or environment required: A large, comfortable room and a circle of straight-backed chairs.

Process

1. The facilitator invites each group member to assess their personal weaknesses and strengths and to disclose these to the group.

2. Following this disclosure, the group member invites feedback of perceived weaknesses and strengths from other group members.

Thus, in this stage, the rest of the group tell the individual about their perceptions of that individual.

3. When each member has both offered assessment and received feedback, the facilitator invites a free discussion on the process.

Evaluation

The facilitator may want to ask:

● What were the differences between your assessment of yourself and that of the group?

Notes

The process can also be used at the end of a learning session as a means of self and peer evaluation. It is important that assessment and feedback are always offered in the order:

(a) weaknesses and
(b) strengths,
   so that the process ends on a positive note.

Exercise 50

Aim of the exercise: To close a group.
Group size: Any number from 6 to 20.
Time required: 10 minutes.
Materials and/or environment required: A large, comfortable room and a circle of straight-backed chairs.

Process

1. The facilitator invites the group to stand up, to move into a close, standing circle and to put their arms around the shoulders of the people standing next to them.
2. Group members are then encouraged to share thoughts about the days activities or about each other.
3. After a few minutes, the group disbands without further discussion.

Exercises in group facilitation

The term 'facilitator' has been used throughout this section of the book to described the person who initiates group activity or who leads the group in some way. The lecturer or tutor running such a group, whose aim is developing self-awareness is a facilitator, as is the student nurses who sets up a learning group for patients in a clinical setting. The nurse who acts as facilitator needs to make some considerations about how to fulfil that role prior to setting up the group in question.

Facilitator style

John Heron (1977c) has described six dimensions of what he calls 'facilitator style' that may help here. Those dimensions are outlined in Fig. 5.4. It is not suggested that a potential facilitator must use one particular aspect of a dimension rather than another but rather that such a decision will arise out of the *type* of group that is to be facilitated. The analysis of facilitator styles is particularly useful in identifying the *range* of possible options open to the group leader.

The sorts of questions that may be asked in relation to the six dimension before attempting to facilitate a group are as follows:

1. Does this group need to be *led* or can it be free flowing and open ended (the directive-non-directive dimension).
2. Do I need to explain what is happening in the group? Do I need to offer theories and frameworks for understanding what is going on or can the group 'explain itself'? (the interpretative-non-interpretative dimension).
3. Do I need to challenge the group and to point out rigidities and repetitions in group and individual behaviour or can I let the group sorts these issues out for themselves (the confronting-non-confronting dimension).
4. Will I be able to handle the expression of laughter, tears, anger or fear or will I need to divert it through lighter topics (the cathartic-non-cathartic dimension).
5. Should I use exercises, games, plans and set procedures to bring structure to the group or should I let the group organize itself? (the structuring-unstructuring dimension).
6. Am I going to let the group share my own thoughts and feelings

1. **Directive**
   The facilitator
   clearly directs
   the group

   or

   Non-directive
   The facilitator
   encourages the
   group to make
   decisions for
   itself.

2. **Interpretative**
   The faciliator
   offers the group
   interpretations of its
   behaviour

   or

   Non-interpretative
   The facilitator
   encourages the
   group to interpret
   its own behaviour

3. **Confronting**
   The facilitator
   challenges the group

   or

   Non-confronting
   The facilitator
   encourages the
   group to challenge
   itself.

4. **Cathartic**
   The facilitator
   encourages the
   release of emotions
   in the group

   or

   Non-cathartic
   The facilitator
   steers the group
   into less emotional
   territory

5. **Structuring**
   The facilitator
   uses activities,
   exercises and games
   to bring structure
   to the group

   or

   Un-structuring
   The facilitator
   works with the group
   in a less formal way

6. **Disclosing**
   The facilitator
   shares his/her
   own thoughts,
   feelings and
   experiences
   with the group

   or

   Non-disclosing
   The facilitator
   keeps his/her own
   thoughts, feelings
   and experiences
   to herself

Fig. 5.4   *Dimensions of facilitator style (after Heron, 1989b)*

as the occur or will I play a more neutral role? (the disclosing-non-disclosing dimension).

Sometimes the *aim and purpose* of the group meeting will help to determine the style to be used. Consider, for example, the following types of groups. What would be examples of *inappropriate* styles of group facilitation in each one?

● a planning meeting
● a group therapy meeting
● a meeting of friends in the pub
● a political meeting
● a discussion group in the school or college

The nurse, lecturer, tutor or trainer who considers these issues is developing the conscious use of self alluded to earlier. If these issues are clarified the facilitator will be in a better position to act knowingly rather that blindly or unawarely. We cannot *change* our behaviour until we *know* what our behaviour is. To go to a group prepared in this way is to have considered the needs of the group. Not all groups are the same and not all groups will require the same sorts of facilitation.

Generally, a useful rule for working with self-awareness groups is to begin with a directive, structured and lightly confronting approach and to gradually help the group to take more and more responsibility for itself. As the group progresses, the facilitator is, on the one hand, increasingly non-directive, unstructuring and non-confronting and on the other, increasingly cathartic and disclosing. Whether or not to be interpretative of other people's behaviour is a moot point. As a rule (and adopting a phenomenological point of view) such interpretations are probably best left to the individual to make. It is often better to be *descriptive* rather than interpretative. This difference is demonstrated as follows:

> A group is discussing a point which causes one member to begin to move around in his or her seat and to stop talking. The group facilitator who is being *descriptive* says: 'I notice that you are quieter than you were and that you are shifting around in your seat quite at lot.' The group facilitator who is *interpretative* says: 'I think you are finding this discussion a bit difficult and that it is making you anxious'.
> The description allows group members to interpret

their own behaviour and to report their own feelings
as they choose. The interpretation pre-empts the
individuals perception of what they are doing and
why they are doing it.

Figure 5.5 summarizes these points about the changing emphasis of
group facilitation.

The general points that may be made about the nurse, tutor,
lecturer or trainer who is facilitating a well-established group is that
he or she should not over-direct the group but should allow it to
develop for itself. Facilitators should not depend too much on structured exercises but allow the group to develop its own structure.
They should consider allowing the free expression of emotion
where it is appropriate and not be prepared to rush in a try to rescue
or 'explain' people's emotions to them. They should not rush to
interpret other people's behaviour but encourage individuals to
make their own sense of what happens to them. These points are
generally in line with the philosophy of experiential learning so far
discussed (although the list contains rather too may 'shoulds' and

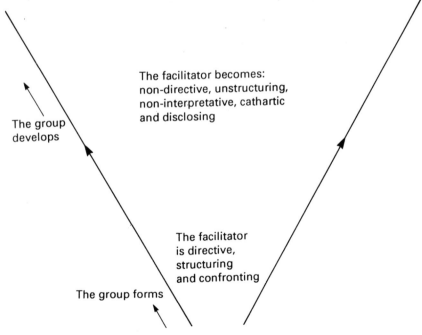

Fig. 5.5 *Appropriate styles of group facilitation for self-awareness groups*

'nots' for my liking!). Experiential learning is, after all, about the reflection on personal experience and about the personal ownership and transformation of meaning. We can never create meaning for other people: in the end each person finds it for themself.

The exercises that follow allow for a systematic investigation of the six dimensions of facilitator style. They may be used progressively and in order so that a range of facilitation skills is built up. Alternatively, one or two may be selected to develop a particular aspect of facilitation. As with Heron's (1989a) Six Category Intervention Analysis (out of which the dimensions were developed), the skilled facilitator is one who can freely choose and intelligently use any aspect of the six dimensions.

It is possible to combine the use of the styles of facilitation with the skills learned through the use of Six Category Intervention Analysis. Figure 5.6 illustrates the relationship between these two models. The styles of facilitation model outlines the general considerations that a group facilitator must make: the category analysis equips them with a range of specific *group interventions*.

In the end, both the styles model and the category analysis have wide application in teaching and learning, nursing practice, organising and running meetings, clinical supervision, research supervision and the development of interpersonal or human skills.

Exercise 51

Aim of the exercise: To exercise a directive style of group facilitation.

Group size: Any number from 6 to 20.

Time required: About 1 hour.

Materials and/or environment required: A large, comfortable room and a circle of straight-backed chairs.

Process

1. The facilitator decides upon a subject for discussion by the group and keeps the group to the topic.
2. After half an hour the facilitator sums up and closes the discussion.

STAGE ONE: SETTING UP A GROUP

Question: What *general* considerations do I need to make about group facilitation before I start running a group?

Answer: Consult dimensions of facilitator style and choose from the following dimensions:

Directive style _____	Non-directive style
Interpretative style _____	Non-interpretative style
Confronting style _____	Non-confronting style
Cathartic style _____	Non-cathartic style
Structuring style _____	Un-structuring style
Disclosing style _____	Non-disclosing style

Consider, also:

1. Stages of group formation
   —forming
   —storming
   —norming
   —performing

2. Group dynamics:
   —pairing
   —rescuing
   —scapegoating etc.

3. Environmental considerations:
   —seating
   —lighting
   —ventilation, etc.

↓   ↓   ↓

STAGE TWO; FACILITATING THE GROUP

Question: What *specific* interventions can I make when I facilitate the group?

Answer: Consult six category intervention analysis and choose from the following interventions:

- Prescriptive interventions
- Informative interventions
- Confronting interventions
- Cathartic interventions
- Catalytic interventions
- Supportive interventions

Fig. 5.6 *The relationship between the dimensions of facilitator style and six category intervention analysis*

3. Facilitators self–evaluate their own performance by describing the shortcomings and strengths of their facilitation to their group.

4. Facilitator invite peer evaluation by asking for feedback from the group on their performance. It is helpful if group members first

say what they *did not like* about their facilitation and then what they *liked* about it.

Notes

In this and all the activities designed to exercise particular facilit-ation skills, the term 'facilitator' can either mean the tutor, lecturer or other nursing professional or it can refer to the student in a group who is learning to facilitate groups.

Exercise 52

Aim of the exercise: To exercise a non-directive style of group facilitation.
Group size: Any number from 6 to 20.
Time required: About 1 hour.
Materials and/or environment required: A large, comfort-able room and a circle of straight-backed chairs.

Process

1. The facilitator asks the group what they would like to talk about and allows a free ranging discussion to develop, making no attempt to keep the group to the topic but allowing the discussion to evolve as the group wishes. Facilitators should try to restrict their interventions to the following:

    ● open questions
    ● reflections
    ● empathy building statements

2. After half an hour the facilitator closes the discussion without summary.
3. Facilitators self-evaluate their own performance by describing the shortcomings and strengths of their facilitation to the group.
4. Facilitator invites peer evaluation by asking for feedback from the group on their performance. It is helpful if group members first say what they *did not like* about the facilitation and then what they *liked* about it.

Exercise 53

Aim of the exercise: To exercise an interpretative style of group facilitation.
Group size: Any number from 6 to 20.
Time required: About 1 hour.
Materials and/or environment required: A large, comfortable room and a circle of straight-backed chairs.

Process

1. The facilitator either decides on a topic for discussion or negotiates a topic with the group.
2. During the discussion, the facilitator offers possible explanations for the behaviour, ideas or feelings of group members.
3. After half an hour, the facilitator sums up both the content of the group discussion and attempts to shed light on the process that occurred.
4. Facilitator self-evaluate their own performance by describing the shortcomings and strengths of the facilitation to the group.
5. Facilitator invites peer evaluation by asking for feedback from the group on his or their performance. It is helpful if group members first say what they *did not like* about the facilitation and then what they *liked* about it.

Notes

The facilitator may want to choose from a variety of theoretical frameworks from which to interpret the groups behaviour, thoughts, feelings or ideas. A short list of such theoretical frameworks might include:

- psychodynamic theory
- behavioural theory
- humanistic theory
- sociological theory
- theological theory
- transactional analalytic theory
- gestalt theory
  etc.

The problem with this approach is whether or not the facilitator ever knows enough about a theoretical framework to make an informed interpretation. Thus the accent in the text, above, on inviting the group members to make sense of *their own* experience wherever possible. A central tenet of this book is that we are the experts on our own behaviour, thoughts and feelings.

Exercise 54

Aim of the exercise: To exercise a non-interpretative style of group facilitation.
Group size: Any number from 6 to 20.
Time required: About 1 hour.
Materials and/or environment required: A large, comfortable room and a circle of straight-backed chairs.

Process

1. The facilitator either decides upon a topic for discussion or negotiates the topic with the group.
2. During the discussion, the facilitator invites possible explanations for the behaviour, thoughts, feelings or ideas from the group members. The facilitator pays particular attention to group members interpretations of *their own* behaviour, thoughts and feelings. The facilitators offer no interpretation of their own but can report to the group on *their own* thoughts and feelings.
3. After half an hour, the facilitator draws the discussion to a close and invites the group to sum up the main issues that have been discussed.
4. Facilitators self-evaluate their own performance by describing the shortcomings and strengths of the facilitation to the group.
5. The facilitator invites peer evaluation by asking for feedback from the group on her performance. It is helpful if group members first say what they *did not like* about her facilitation and then what they *liked* about it.

Exercise 55

Aim of the exercise: To exercise a confronting style of group facilitation.
Group size: Any number from 6 to 20.
Time required: About 1 hour.
Materials and/or environment required: A large, comfortable room and a circle of straight-backed chairs.

Process

1. The facilitator either decides upon a topic for discussion or negotiates a topic with the group.
2. During the discussion, the facilitator draws attention to any of the following:

   - errors of logic in a group members' argument,
   - mismatches between what group members are *saying* and their facial expression or 'body language',
   - repetitions,
   - errors of fact
   - any tendency for a group member to generalise from a single case,
   - a silent member of the group

3. After half an hour the facilitator draws the discussion to a close and sums up the content and process of the discussion.
4. Facilitators self-evaluate their own performance by describing the shortcomings and strengths of their facilitation to the group.
5. Facilitator invite peer evaluation by asking for feedback from the group on their performance. It is helpful if group members first say what they *did not like* about the facilitation and then what they *liked* about it.

Exercise 56

Aim of the exercise: To exercise a non-confronting style of group leadership.
Group size: Any number from 6 to 20.

Time required: About 1 hour.
Materials and/or environment required: A large, comfortable room and a circle of straight-backed chairs.

Process

1. The facilitator either decides upon a topic for discussion or negotiates a topic with the group.
2. Before commencing the discussion, the facilitator invites the group to be awake to the occurrence of any errors of logic, repetitive behaviour, contradictions and so forth.
3. During the discussion, the facilitator makes no attempt to confront the group or individual members but allows the group to make its own confrontations.
4. Facilitators self-evaluate their own performance by describing the shortcomings and strengths of their facilitation to the group.
5. Facilitators invite peer evaluation by asking for feedback from the group on their performance. It is helpful if group members first say what they *did not like* about their facilitation and then what they *liked* about it.

Notes

It is often a good idea to run these activities one after the other as a series of pairs. Thus, the confronting activity is followed by the non-confronting activity, both lead by the same person. Following a pair or exercises, both the facilitator and the group can decide which style they prefer and suggest when one style would be more appropriately used than the other.

Exercise 57

Aim of the exercise: To exercise a cathartic style of group facilitation.
Group size: Any number from 6 to 20.
Time required: About 2 hours.
Materials and/or environment required: A large, comfortable room and a circle of straight-backed chairs.

Process

1. The facilitator invites the group to embark on a discussion about personal or emotional issues. Clearly such a topic must be negotiated with the group.
2. The facilitator makes it clear at the outset that group members are free to express any feelings as they occur.
3. During the discussion, the facilitator tries to restrict his or her interventions to the following:

   - he or she invites particular group members to literally describe a place that they have been talking about that seems to evoke emotion,
   - the facilitator asks particular group members to note how they are feeling and to *exaggerate* the way that they are feeling,
   - the facilitator encourages particular group members to exaggerate hand movements and gestures that they make and then asks ... 'What's the feeling that goes with that ...?'

4. After about three quarters of an hour, the facilitator draws the discussion to a close and to a lighter level as necessary. Such lightening of the atmosphere may be achieved by one of the following mini exercises:
   (a) each person in turn describes something that they are looking forward to,
   (b) each person in turn describes his or her house, car or some other fairly 'neutral' object.
5. Facilitators self-evaluate their own performance by describing the shortcomings and strengths of their facilitation to the group.
6. Facilitators invite peer evaluation by asking for feedback from the group on their performance. It is helpful if group members first say what they *did not like* about their facilitation and then what they *liked* about it.

Notes

It is recommended that the group facilitator who wishes to develop a wide range of cathartic skills considers undergoing specific training in them. Training courses in managing other people's emotions are often offered by colleges, polytechnics and university departments, particularly those with an interest in humanistic psychology and 'growth' work.

Exercise 58

Aim of the exercise: To exercise a non-cathartic style of group facilitation.
Group size: Any number from 6 to 20.
Time required: About 1 hour.
Materials and/or environment required: A large, comfortable room and a circle of straight-backed chairs.

Process

1. The facilitator either decides on a topic for discussion or negotiates a topic with the group.
2. During the discussion that follows, the facilitator purposely avoids issues that are emotionally charged and if emotional issues do arise, deflects them by moving the discussion onto a lighter level.
3. After half an hour the facilitator draws the discussion to a close and summarizes the content and process of the discussion as necessary.
4. Facilitators self-evaluate their own performance by describing the shortcomings and strengths of their facilitation to the group.
5. Facilitators invite peer evaluation by asking for feedback from the group on their performance. It is helpful if group members first say what they *did not like* about the facilitation and then what they *liked* about it.

Notes

The skill of moving between levels of emotion in group work is an important one. Even when a contract has been drawn up with a particular group that allows the expression of emotion, it is important the facilitator does not 'hound' the group or overstate the need for emotional release. The facilitator who can use a light approach, even with heavyweight topics is likely to be more successful that the one who is always earnest and meaningful in her approach. Paradoxically, the light approach can often allow for a far greater expression of emotion that can the 'earnest' approach.

Exercise 59

Aim of the exercise: To exercise a structuring style of group facilitation.

Group size: Any number from 6 to 20.

Time required: Between 1 and 2 hours.

Materials and/or environment required: A large, comfortable room and a circle of straight-backed chairs.

Process

1. The facilitator introduces and explains the rules of a structured exercise or activity to the group. One from the earlier part of this chapter may be used. Others are described by Kagan, Evans and Kay (1986).
2. The group undertakes the exercise and the facilitator pays close attention to giving clear instructions and keeps a close eye on timing.
3. The facilitator invites the group to reconvene after the exercise and asks each member of the group to complete the following two sentences:
   (a) 'What I liked least about this exercise was ...'
   (b) 'What I liked best about this exercise was ...'
4. Facilitators self-evaluates their own performance by describing the shortcomings and strengths of their facilitation to the group.
5. Facilitators invites peer evaluation by asking for feedback from the group on their performance. It is helpful if group members first say what they *did not like* about their facilitation and then what they *liked* about it.

Notes

It has been noted, above, that it is often a good idea to *start* a series of group meetings with plenty of structure. Too little can make the meetings seem aimless. Structure can easily be dropped as the group develops a sense of identity. On the other hand, it is often difficult to *introduce* structure if it has not been there previously.

Exercise 60

Aim of the exercise: To exercise an unstructuring style of group facilitation.
Group size: Any number from 6 to 20.
Time required: About 1 hour.
Materials and/or environment required: A large, comfortable room and a circle of straight-backed chairs.

Process

1. The facilitator invites suggestions from the group as to any exercises, games etc. that the group would like to undertake.
2. The facilitator, may, as required, invite a member of the group to take over group facilitation for the exercise.
3. Alternatively, the facilitator helps the group to undertake the exercise but remains an almost equal member of the group and does not try to impose any structure on what is happening.
4. After the activity has been completed, the facilitators self-evaluate their own performance by describing the shortcomings and strengths of their facilitation to the group.
5. Facilitator invite peer evaluation by asking for feedback from the group on their performance. It is helpful if group members first say what they *did not like* about the facilitation and then what they *liked* about it.

Exercise 61

Aim of the exercise: To explore lack of structure in a group setting.
Group size: Any number from 6 to 20.
Time required: About 1½ hours.
Materials and/or environment required: A large, comfortable room and a circle of straight-backed chairs.

Process

1. The facilitator walks into the group, sits down and remains silent for the duration of an hour. They allow the group to unfold (or not) as it will.

2. At the end of the hour they declare the exercise complete and invokes a discussion on the experience.

3. The facilitator self-evaluates their own performance by describing the shortcomings and strengths of their facilitation to the group.

4. The facilitator invites peer evaluation by asking for feedback from the group on their performance. It is helpful if group members first say what they *did not like* about the facilitation and then what they *liked* about it.

Notes

This is the extreme example of an unstructuring approach. A similar approach, from a therapeutic point of view is described by Bion (1961) in his classic book on running groups. Often, the following stages may be observed with this activity:

(a) the group is confused and sometimes amused by what is happening,

(b) several, usually abortive attempts are made to take over leadership and begin an activity,

(c) the groups get angry with the facilitators for not carrying out their 'proper' role,

(d) the group ignore the facilitators and attempt to carry on as though the facilitators were not there.

This format requires a certain bravery on the part of the facilitator (and on the part of the group!) but it can be a useful way of exploring issues of dependency and independence.

Exercise 62

Aim of the exercise: To exercise a disclosing style of group facilitation.

Group size: Any number from 6 to 20.

Time required: About 1 hour.
Materials and/or environment required: A large, comfortable room and a circle of straight-backed chairs.

Process

1. The facilitator shares a story, anecdote or personal experience with the group and develops a discussion based on it.
2. During the discussion the facilitator shares his or her immediate and/or past experiences with group members.
3. After three quarters of an hour, the facilitator sums up the content and process of the group as required, or invites the group members to do so.
4. The facilitator self-evaluates his or her own performance by describing the shortcomings and strengths of her facilitation to the group.
5. The facilitator invites peer evaluation by asking for feedback from the group on her performance. It is helpful if group members first say what they *did not like* about the facilitation and then what they *liked* about it.

Exercise 63

Aim of the exercise: To exercise a non-disclosing style of group leadership.
Group size: Any number from 6 to 20.
Time required: About 1 hour.
Materials and/or environment required: A large, comfortable room and a circle of straight-backed chairs.

Process

1. The facilitator invites stories, anecdotes or experiences from the group and develops a discussion around them.
2. During the discussion that follows facilitators encourage the sharing of experiences by members of the group but at no point discloses their own feelings or thoughts. They deflect any direct questions from group members.

3. After half and hour, the facilitator draws the discussion to a close and sums up the content and process of the activity as required.
4. The facilitator self-evaluates her own performance by describing the shortcomings and strengths of their facilitation to the group.
5. The facilitator invites peer evaluation by asking for feedback from the group on the performance. It is helpful if group members first say what they *did not like* about the facilitation and then what they *liked* about it.

Notes

'Disclosure begets disclosure' (Jourard 1964). The disclosing facilitator can often encourage the group to talk more freely and easily once they realize that the facilitator is also prepared to give of themself. On the other hand, it is easy to *over disclose*. The facilitator who discloses too much, too quickly is likely to alienate themself from the group who think: 'Am *I* going to have to reveal *myself* in this way?' Judging levels of disclosure is a fairly precise business.

Recording and Evaluating Group Work

It is often helpful to know how a group is changing as it works together. One very simple format for checking, verbally, on progress in the group is to ask at the end of a session or a day for the group to work through two 'rounds'. During the first round, each person in turn completes the sentence: 'What I liked least about this session was ...'. When everybody has completed the statement, a second round is completed using the sentence: 'What I like most about this session was ...'. This offers a quick and subjective method of evaluation. Another approach is to hold a short 'unfinished business' session at the end of each day. Ten minutes is left at the end in which anyone is free to say anything, positive or negative about the day. They are free to surface any doubts, annoyances, pleasant experiences—anything. They may also want to say something to another member of the group that up to that point they had only been thinking. The idea behind this 'air clearing' activity is that it is probably as well to verbalise some of these thoughts and feelings that are just below the surface rather than to carry them out of the

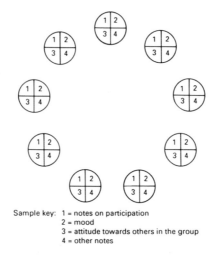

Sample key: 1 = notes on participation
             2 = mood
             3 = attitude towards others in the group
             4 = other notes

Fig. 5.7   *A format for recording group progress (after Cox, 1978)*

group. During the unfinished business session, the facilitator does not respond to the statements that are made other than by accepting them.

Another, more permanent method of charting progress is through the use of a visual device such as the one developed out of Cox's (1978) work (Fig 5.7). Each circle represents one of the group members. Each circle can be divided up in any way that the facilitator finds useful and each segment of the circle can then be used to record notes about each member of the group. A fresh sheet record sheet is kept for each meeting of the group and the collected sheets serves as an evaluation device.

An alternative to this is that the circles are drawn on a large sheet of paper and group members record their feelings and thoughts at the end of each session. The sheets are then kept for display whilst subsequent meetings are in progress.

Other methods of assessment, both objective and subjective may be used to chart educational progress if the focus of the group is mainly and educational or training one. Neil Kenworthy and Peter Nicklin offer an excellent review of up-to-date assessment methods (Kenworthy and Nicklin 1989).

Through the series of exercises in group membership and group facilitation described in this chapter can be developed skills that may be carried over into any nursing situation. That they *are* carried over is a fundamental issue. Clearly, any amount of group work in the context of nursing is of little value if it does not lead to a positive change in nursing practice. Sometimes the transfer of learning takes place at a subtle level: the nurse modifies her attitudes or takes more notice of what they do and say. Sometimes the change is quite clear and nursing students begin to set up groups and run them effectively. It is important, though, that constant reference to nursing is made during training sessions that incorporate the exercises in this chapter.

Finally, an outline programme for a workshop on group facilitation skills is offered that can be adapted for use in any nurse education or training course.

A programme for group facilitation training

1. Introductions
   (a) The group facilitator introduces the aims of the workshop and outlines domestic arrangements; meal breaks and tea and coffee breaks.
   (b) the facilitator invites the group members to introduce themselves using the approach outlined in this book. Icebreakers can also be used as required.
   (c) the facilitator discusses the aims of the workshop and introduces the two principles:
       (i) the voluntary principle: that everyone is free to take part in activities or to sit out of them as they see fit,
       (ii) the proposal clause: that group members should take responsibility for suggesting that the group either spends more time on a certain section of the workshop or that things are speeded up.
2. Theory Input
   (a) The facilitator offers a short theory input on group theory and group dynamics
   (b) The group undertake one or two group memberships exercises (e.g. exercises 30–50 from this book).
   (c) The facilitator introduces the concept of Dimensions of Facilitator Styles and discusses these with the group.
3. Experiential learning activities
   (a) Individual members of the group take turns in leading the

group by working with different styles of group facilitation (Exercises 51-63 in this book).

(b) Volunteers then lead the group for longer periods (between 1 and 2 hours using either one particular style or using an eclectic style incorporating many different aspects of the dimensions of facilitator styles. The later choice is not a good one early on in a course as it is often difficult for group members (and the facilitator) to determine what style is being used at any given time.

(c) The volunteers from (b), above, self evaluate their facilitation skills in front of the group and invite feedback from the group and from the facilitator of the workshop.

4. Evaluation and application

(a) a final plenary session is held to discuss the application of the new skills to the clinical or community setting.

(b) the facilitator leads a evaluation session and closes the workshop.

This format can be adapted for use as a one or two day workshop, a week long workshop or as a series of study days.

6

Experiential Exercises for Human Skills—Self-awareness Methods

> The idea expressed in the Biblical 'love they neighbour as thyself' implies that respect for one's own integrity and uniqueness, love for and understanding of one's own self, cannot be separated from respect and love and understanding for another individual. The love for my own self is inseparably connected with love for any other being (Fromm, 1975).
>
> We are what we pretend to be—so take care what you pretend to be (Vonnegut, 1968).

The last two chapters explored a range of exercises that develop self-awareness related to counselling and group skills. This chapter offers other activities that may be used to further self-awareness. They will enhance interpersonal contact in both one-to-one and group situations. Some may be undertaken alone: others need a group setting. The experiential learning cycle should be adhered to as with the preceding exercises. That is to say that after a particular activity has been undertaken, some time should be allowed for both reflection on the experience and for future planning about how the learning gained can be applied to the practical nursing situation. Sometimes such links are clear, sometimes they are not immediately obvious. If time is taken in this reflective and planning stage, more benefit is likely to be experienced.

Some of the methods here are related to meditation, relaxation and body-awareness. All of them can be repeated and some are, at first, difficult. Repeating the exercises a number of times over a period of weeks can bring particular and lasting changes in self-awareness. No attempt is made to develop a particular theoretical framework around these exercises and activities. The titles at the end of this book offer a variety of theoretical viewpoints on many of the exercises contained here.

The serious student of meditation and stress reduction is recommended to refer to the considerable literature on these particular fields in order to take their studies further. The exercises, alone, however, can serve as valuable means of becoming more relaxed. They also help to develop a heightened sense of body awareness and mind—including the thoughts, feelings, sensations and intuitions discussed earlier in this book.

It is quite possible to tailor many of these activities (and, indeed, the exercises in previous chapters) either to suit yourself or to suit the group that you are facilitating or are a member of. Often the activities that you think up on the spur of the moment are just the ones that suit the group at that particular time. It is also helpful if students who are group members are encouraged to bring new activities to the group. It is also an aid to developing group skills if those students are encouraged to facilitate the group during the activity. They may want to run a whole morning, afternoon or day's activities or to organize only the running of the activity. Either way, it is helpful if all of the stages of the experiential learning cycle are worked through. As we noted earlier, it is usually the reflective stage that is rushed and yet this is arguably the stage in which most learning is likely to occur.

Exploring Self Concept

Exercise 64

Aim of the exercise: To explore self concept.
Group size: This activity can be carried out by the person working on her own or by a small group of up to 10 people.
Time required: Between ½ hour and 2 hours.
Materials required: Paper and pen.

Process

On a piece of paper, write a description of yourself in the *third person*. In other words, write about yourself as if you were describing another person. Your account will tend to start as follows:

> 'Jane Smith is a girl who lives ...' or

'Andrew is a staff nurse working in a large district
general hospital ...'

Write in this way for as long as you can and cover as many aspects
of yourself as you can. If you get stuck, stop and begin a new para-
graph, starting from a different aspect of yourself.

Evaluation

Read through what you have written. What do you notice about
what you have put down on paper? Is the 'you' described in writing
the 'you' that you imagine yourself to be or are there some surprises?

Notes

You may like to try this exercise with another person whom you
know fairly well. You may also then write a piece *about each other* and
compare the differences in accounts.

This activity has been used in both therapy and research and a
fuller version of the approach is described by Bannister and Fransella (1986).

Exercise 65

Aim of the exercise: To explore a changing sense of self.
Group size: This activity can be carried out by the person
working on their own or by a small group of up to 10 people.
Time required: Between ½ hour and 2 hours.
Materials required: Paper and pen.

Process

1. Use the following headings on four separate sheets of paper:
   (a) (your name) ... ten years ago,
   (b) (your name) ... five years ago,
   (c) (your name) ... now,
   (d) (your name) as I would like to be in the future.
2. Fill in the sheets with accounts of yourself according the headings
   on each sheet. Write as much as you can and don't pay attention
   to style, punctuation and so forth. The aim should be to write
   as quickly and as fluently as you can.

3. When you have completed the activity, read through the sheets and compare the word portraits that you have written.

Evaluation

If this activity is carried out in a group the facilitator may want to 'process' the activity in one of the ways described in the previous chapter. It is important that no one is forced to disclose things about themselves that they would rather keep private.

Exercise 66

Aim of the exercise: To explore personal feelings and beliefs about the self.
Group size: Any number from 6 to 20.
Time required: About 1½ hours.
Materials and/or environment required: A large, comfortable room and a circle of straight-backed chairs. A handout prepared from material below.

Process

1. The facilitator gives out a handout containing the words listed below.
2. Each person works through the list and identifies the words that he or she feels best describes his or herself.
3. The group is invited to pair off and to discuss their findings with a partner.
4. After 20 minutes the group is reconvened and a discussion is held on how we develop a sense of self.

The words are:

Concerned	Caring	Impulsive
Secretive	Friendly	Lonely
Thoughtful	Disagreeable	Reliable
Shy	Depressive	Solitary
Aggressive	Cheerful	Antagonistic
Moody	Attractive	Awkward
Skilful	Mean	

Evaluation:

The facilitator may want to ask:

- How do you *know* these things are true about you?
- What has contributed to your being this way?
- Did you agree with your partners' assessments of themselves?
- How would you assess them differently?

Professional Values Questionnaire

Exercise 67

Aim of the exercise: To examine professional values.
Group size: Any number from 6 to 20.
Time required: About 2 hours.
Materials and/or environment required: A large, comfortable room and a circle of straight-backed chairs. A handout (Fig 6.1).

Professional Values Questionnaire

Read each of the following statments and circle either A, if you agree with the statement or B if you disagree with it.

1. Abortion should be available on demand.	A	B
2. People should always be told if they are dying.	A	B
3. People have a right to refuse life-saving treatment.	A	B
4. I should be allowed to refuse to work with people who have AIDS.	A	B
5. I would always report a senior colleague whom I knew to be taking drugs from the medicine trolley.	A	B
6. People's religious beliefs should always be respected.	A	B
7. Terminally ill people should have the right to end their own lives.	A	B
8. Gay partners should be able to be considered as next of kin.	A	B
9. Suicide is wrong in all cases.	A	B
10. Patients should be allowed to read their case notes on request.	A	B

Fig. 6.1 *A personal values questionnaire for use with exercise 67.*

Process

1. The facilitator gives out the following handout to the group and asks them to consider each statement and to mark alongside each statement whether or not they agree or disagree with each item. They should try to avoid marking 'don't know'.
2. After ten minutes, the facilitator invites the group to break into pairs to discuss their responses.
3. After a further ten minutes, the facilitator reconvenes the group and invokes a discussion on the issues that are raised.

Evaluation

The facilitator may want to ask:

- How did you develop your professional values?
- Are there legal implications for any of the statements?
- Could you ever *change* your values?
- What might influence you to change them?

Notes

This type of exercise is similar to those known as values clarification activities (Simon, Howe and Kirschenbaum 1978; Steel and Harmon, 1983). Such activities are an important means of exploring core values. Arguably, it is our values that shape our behaviour and that, in turn, effect our nursing practice.

Meditation

Meditation has been used for centuries for mystical, religious and secular purposes. There are many excellent accounts of the history and theory behind various meditational practices (see, for examples: Tart, 1969; Le Shan, 1974; Hewitt, 1978; Pierce, 1982; Bond, 1986). The following activities are simple and effective. They can be used to explore self-awareness or they can be used simply as a means of inducing relaxation. They can be used by the individual or by a small group. They are described as though they relate to the individual meditating on his or her own. If they are used in a small group setting, it is advisable to find a room where people can be undisturbed and quiet. It is also probably better if the facilitator does not try too hard at invoking a 'mysterious' atmosphere.

Exercise 68

Aim of the exercise: To practice the meditational process of 'counting the breaths'.
Group size: May be practised alone or with others.
Time required: Periods starting from 2 minutes and building up to half an hour, twice a day.
Materials and/or environment required: A quiet place where distractions of noise, interruptions and os on are within a tolerable level. The meditator may sit on the floor or in a straight-backed chair.

Process

1. Sit motionless, comfortably and with the eyes closed.
2. Breath quietly and gently. Breath in through the nostrils and out through the mouth.
3. Let your attention focus on your breathing.
4. Begin to count your breaths, from 1–10. One is the whole cycle of an inhalation and an exhalation. Two is the next complete cycle.
5. When the breaths have been counted from 1–10, begin to count the next set from 1–10 and so on.
6. If you are distracted or lose count, simply go back to the beginning and start again.

Notes

In the early stages of meditation, it is very easy to be distracted by what Pearce calls 'roof-brain' chatter (Pearce, 1982), the seemingly endless flow of thoughts and ideas that refuse to go away when we sit down to meditation. Meditation, like most things, take practice and commitment. Slowly, the 'roof-brain' chatter dies away.

Exercise 69

Aim of the exercise: To practice the meditational process of internal witnessing.

Group size: May be practised alone or with others.
Time required: Periods starting with two minutes and building up to ½ hour, twice a day.
Materials and/or environment required: A quiet place where distractions of noise, interruptions and so on are within a tolerable level. The meditator may sit on the floor or in a straight-backed chair. An object of contemplation; the flame of a candle, a flower, a picture, an ornament etc.

Process

1. Sit motionless in front of the object of contemplation.
2. Breath quietly and gently. Breath in through the nostrils and out through the mouth.
3. Let your attention focus on the object of contemplation. Concentrate on it and allow it to be the only focus of your attention.
4. If you are distracted, gently bring your attention back to the object.

Exercise 70

Aim of the exercise: To experience complete relaxation.
Group size: This activity can be carried out by the person on his or her own or in the company of a small group.
Time required: About 40 minutes.
Materials and/or environment required: A large, comfortable room in which the person or persons can lie on the floor.

Process

1. The participants lie on the floor with plenty of space between them.
2. The following script is read by the facilitator at normal speed in a quiet but not 'hypnotic' voice.

'Lie on your back, with your hands by your sides ... stretch your legs out and have your feet about a foot apart ... Pay attention to your breathing ... take two or three really deep breaths ... now allow

your head to sink into the floor … your head is sinking into the floor and you begin to feel more and more relaxed … allow your brow to become smooth and relaxed … feel your cheeks relaxing … let your jaw drop and relax … feel the tension draining out of your temples as your jaw relaxes … let yourself relax … more and more … let your shoulders drop and feel your neck and shoulders relax … more and more relaxed … now become aware of your right arm … let your right arm become heavy and warm and relaxed … your upper right arm … lower arm … your right hand … the whole of your right arm is heavy and warm and relaxed … no tension … just relaxed … now become aware of your left arm … let your left arm become heavy and warm and relaxed … your upper left arm … lower arm … your left hand feels heavy and warm and relaxed … the whole of your left arm is heavy and warm and relaxed … your shoulders and chest feel relaxed … your abdomen feels relaxed … your pelvis and hips … you're feeling heavy and warm and relaxed … your right leg and foot feels heavy and relaxed … your left leg feels the same … your whole body is relaxed … no tension … just relaxed … and you can appreciate what it feels like to feel safe and warm and relaxed … just lay back and enjoy the feeling … … … …
Now, slowly, stretch yourself … stretch your arms and legs …your toes and fingers … now slowly sit up … taking your time … slowly sit up and take a few deep breaths … and appreciate what it feels like to feel really relaxed.'

Notes

There are numerous variations on this activity and many are described in the literature (see, for example, Bond 1986, Bailey and Clarke, 1989). This activity can be recorded onto a tape, preferably by the person who is going to use it. In this way, the person not only hears his or her own voice reading through the script but also hears herself *telling his or herself* to relax. Such an invocation can aid further relaxation, away from the activity itself. From a practical point of view, if you are taping this script and want to stop for a moment, always press the 'pause' button on the tape recorder. If you use the 'stop' button, you are likely to create a distracting 'click' in the middle of your tape.

Guided Fantasy

The following guided fantasy exercise incorporates aspects of meditation and relaxation. It may be used following either a meditation exercise or the use of the relaxation script. It may also be used on its own. As with both meditation and relaxation, it can be used as a means of de-stressing the mind/body. It can also be used be a preliminary exercise in exploring the transpersonal domain (Vaughan, 1984; Wilber, 1983) or what have been called 'altered states of consciousness'. Such methods have also been used in a nursing and therapeutic settings and have much in common with 'imagery' (Zahourek, 1988). At a simpler level, such an exercise sometimes helps to put things into perspective, to help us to appreciate our true position in the total nature of things. To appreciate what Claxton calls 'the larger canvas' (Claxton, 1984). It may even help in clarifying religious or spiritual beliefs or lack of them. A similar and rather more elaborate version of this exercise is described by Ram Dass (1977).

Exercise 71

Aim of the exercise: To experience relaxation and to explore something different to the normal waking state.
Group size: Any number from 2 to 20.
Time required: About 1 hour.
Materials and/or environment required: A large, comfortable, quiet room in which participants can lay on the floor.

Process

1. The participants undertake the relaxation exercise described above. The activity can also be run from 'cold'.
2. The following script is read by the facilitator at a normal speed in a quiet but not hypnotic voice.

'Lie on your back with your hands by your sides ... stretch your legs out and have your feet about a foot apart ... pay attention to your breathing ... now let your breathing become gentle and relaxed ... now I want you to experience your body growing in size ... your head, your arms, your legs, your trunk ... are all growing in size ... experience that sense of growing and allow yourself to grow more ... experience your growing until your head reaches the top of the ceiling ... feel your vastness ... and experience a feeling of calmness and equanimity ... now continue to grow ... your head goes up into the sky ... until all the surrounding town and countryside is contained within you ... you are continuing to grow ... you grow larger still ... feel you vastness ... until you head is amongst the planets and you are sitting in the middle of the galaxy ... the earth is lying deep inside you ... feel all this and experience the feeling of vastness ... of awe ... of calmness ... sit in this universe ... silent, huge, peaceful ... continue to grow ... until you contain all galaxies ... you are at one with everything ... experience the vastness ... let everything be as it is ... the silence ......

Now, very slowly, allow yourself to return ... come down in size slowly ... past the galaxy ... down, slowly to the size of the earth ... now slowly to the surrounding countryside and towns and notice all that is around you ... now continue to come down in size until you fill the room ... slowly ... gently ... now return to your normal size ... and just lie for a while and experience the sense of peace and relaxation ... think of your experience ... remain quiet and relaxed ... take a couple of deep breaths ... in your own time ... slowly stretch ... sit up gently ... and open your eyes.'

3. After allowing a period of 'coming round', the facilitator invites the group to reconvene and to discuss the experience.

Body-awareness

The exercise in this final section is designed to increase awareness of body perception. It can be used as a means of relaxation and also as a method of becoming more acutely aware of body image, shape and size.

Exercise 72

Aim of the exercise: To explore body image and proprioceptive sense.

Group size: Any number from 2 to 20.

Time required: About 1 hour.
Materials and/or environment required: A large, comfortable room in which participants can lie on the floor.

Process

1. The group members lay on the floor with plenty of space between them.
2. The following script is read by the facilitator at normal speed in a quiet but not hypnotic voice.
   'Lie on your back with your hands by your sides ... stretch your legs out and have your feet about a foot apart ... pay attention to your breathing ... take two or three deep breaths ... now let your breathing become gentle and relaxed ... now I want you to become aware of your body ... starting at the toes ... try to experience the feeling in your feet and toes ... try to experience that as though you were *inside* your feet and toes ... now become aware of the lower parts of your legs ... as if from the inside ... now your knees ... become aware of your joints ... become aware of your thighs and the top of your legs ... experience them as if you were inside them ... now experience you pelvis and hips ... now your abdomen ... as if from the inside ... put your attention into your chest ... experience the feeling inside your chest ... now your hands ... your lower arms ... your upper arms ... imagine being inside your arms ... now experience your shoulders ... feel the shoulder joints ... experience the feeling inside your neck ... the back of your head ... now your head itself ... feel and experience your face ... the muscles in your face ... your lips ... your nose ... your eyes ... finally ... your scalp ... imagine the feeling as though you were beneath your scalp ... remain fully aware of all parts of your body ... notice which parts you can fully experience ... and which parts are numb to you ... see if you can become more aware of those parts of your body ... now just lie and relax for a few more moments ... take a couple of deep breaths ... and slowly ... in your own time ... sit up and open your eyes.

3. After this exercise, the facilitator invites the group to reconvene and initiates a discussion on the experience.

Evaluation

The facilitator may want to ask:

• Which parts of your body did you find to be numb?
• Did you experience any 'gaps' in your experience of your body?

Conclusion

So the series of exercises is complete. The focus of the exercises has shifted from the pair to the group and back to the individual. In closing with the exercises that centre on the self, I emphasizes the theme that has been a recurrent one throughout the book: the development of self-awareness. That self-awareness, however, can never be for its own sake. It is the means by which we differentiate ourselves from other people in order to care for them and help them. If we do not know ourselves, at least to a minimal degree, we are unlikely to be able to help others very much. Without self awareness we will constantly blur the distinction between 'me' and 'you'.

It is hoped that the book offers practical, usable ideas for helping in the development of interpersonal skills and self awareness at all levels in nurse education. The exercises described are only *one* way of doing things. The exercises that you develop yourself can often be just as effective and just as useful.

A programme for self-awareness training

1. Introductions
   (a) The group facilitator introduces the aims of the workshop and outlines domestic arrangements: meal breaks and tea and coffee breaks.
   (b) the facilitator invites the group members to introduce themselves using the approach outlined in this book. Icebreakers can also be used as required.
   (c) the facilitator discusses the aims of the workshop and introduces the two principles:
       (i) the voluntary principle: that everyone is free to take part in activities or to sit out of them as they see fit,
       (ii) the proposal clause: that group members should take responsibility for suggesting that the group either spends more time on a certain section of the workshop or that things are speeded up.

2. Theory Input
   (a) The facilitator offers a short theory input on awareness including inputs on self-concepts, aspects of self and methods of developing self-awareness.
   (b) The group undertake a pairs exercise in which the group pair off and are nominated 'A' and 'B'. 'A' then asks 'B' the question 'Who are you?' 'B' then addresses this question and 'A' repeats the question, twice more, at intervals in order to allow 'B' to readdress it. After ten minutes, roles are reversed and 'B' asks the question, three times, of 'A'. After a further ten minutes, the group facilitator reconvenes the group and facilitates a discussion on the exercise.
3. Experiential Learning Activities
   The group work through a variety of exercises either from this or from previous chapters and plenty of time is allowed, after each, for discussion. A recurrent theme should be: 'how does self-awareness enhance my performance as a nurse?'

Evaluation and Application

(a) a final plenary session is held to discuss the application of the new skills to the clinical or community setting.
(b) the facilitator leads a evaluation session and closes the workshop.

This format can be adapted for use as a one or two day workshop, a week long workshop or as a series of study days.

APPENDIX I

Topics for Pairs Activities

The pairs format described in Chapter 4 is a particularly flexible one for use in the experiential learning mode. The following questions are ones that can be used in that format to explore aspects of self-awareness and interpersonal skills.

These questions can be used in the following way. Members of a learning group pair off and are nominated 'A' and 'B'. 'A' then poses the particular question and listens to 'B''s answer. 'A' then *repeats* the question after two further intervals, so that 'B' can fully explore the question. The activity is not a conversation and 'A''s only task is to listen. After ten minutes, roles are reversed and 'B' poses the question to 'A', three times over a period of ten minutes. When both partners have had their turns, a plenary session is convened.

- What are the personal qualities that make *you* an effective nurse (or counsellor)?
- What do you need to do to become a more effective nurse (or counsellor)?
- How do you look after yourself?
- How do you demonstrate care for others?
- What do you need to do to enhance your care for others?
- What are your best qualities?
- What do others think and feel about you?
- If you had to change some of your personal characteristics, which ones would you change?
- If you had to live in another period in history, which one would you live in ... can you expand on the topic?
- What are your most important beliefs about yourself/your work/your personal life/your relationships?
- What to you need to do to enhance your relationships with others?
- What (if any) spiritual beliefs do you have?
- What have been the most important things that you have learned?
- What would you change about nursing?
- What would you change about other people?
- What sorts of things would you change about society?
- If you were to do something other than nursing, what would it be ... can you expand ...?

- In what ways has nursing changed you?
- What sorts of situations would you find *most difficult* in counselling?
- What sorts of situations would you find *most difficult* in running groups?
- What do you need to do to enhance your facilitation skills?

Topics for Group Activities

Chapter 5 described a range of group activities for use as exploring group membership and group facilitation. The following topics are ones that can be used instead of the suggested ones or as supplementary topics.

- Nurse education and nursing
- Running groups
- Being a nurse counsellor
- Being a group facilitator
- Nursing models and nursing theory
- The theory-practice gap in nursing
- Why do we need self-awareness?
- Stress and nursing
- Problems in running groups
- Problems in being a group member
- Dealing with aggression
- Coping with anxiety
- Our relationships with each other in this group
- The pro's and con's of group activities
- How we've changed as a group
- What we would like to change about the people in this group
- How we are the same as each other and how we differ
- Management and education in nursing
- Difficult patients
- How we could become more assertive
- What we do with our anger
- How we deal with stress
- Socialization into nursing
- How we could be different
- Our beliefs as a group
- What would happen to the group if various members left
- Interpersonal skills training in nursing.

REFERENCES

Alberti R.E., Emmons M.L. (1982). *Your Perfect Right: a Guide to Assertive Living:* 4th edn., San Louis, Impact Publishers.

Alexander F.M. (1969) *Resurrection of the Body:* New York: University Books.

Argyle M. (1975). *The Psychology of Interpersonal Behaviour:* Harmondsworth, Penguin.

Arnold E., Boggs K. (1989). *Interpersonal Relationships: Professional Communication Skills for Nurses:* Philadelphia, PA: Saunders.

Bandler R., Grinder J. (1975). *The Structure of Magic Vol 1: A book about language and therapy:* California: Science and Behaviour Books.

Bannister D., Fransella F. (1986). *Inquiring Man: The Psychology of Personal Constructs:* 3rd Edn, London: Croom Helm.

Bateson C.D., Coke J.S. (1981). Empathy: A source of altruistic motivation for helping? In *Altruism and Helping Behaviour: Social, Personality and Developmental Perspectives. (Rushton J.P., Sorventino R.M. eds.).* New Jersey: Lawrence Erlbaum Associates.

Benson H. (1976). *The Relaxation Response:* London, Collins

Bion W. (1961). *Experiences in Groups:* London, Tavistock.

Blake R.R., Mouton J.S. (1976). *Consultation:* New York, Addison Wesley.

Bond, M. (1986). *Stress and Self-Awareness: a Guide for Nurses:* London: Heinemann.

Bond M. (1987). *Being Assertive: A Distance Learning Pack for Nurses:* London: Distance Learning Centre, South Bank Polytechnic.

Bond M., Kilty J. (1982). *Practical Methods of Coping with Stress, Human Potential Research Project,* Guildford: University of Surrey.

Boore J. (1978). *A Prescription for Recovery:* London: RCN.

Boud D. (ed.) (1981). *Developing Student Autonomy in Learning,* London: Kogan Page.

Boud D. (1989). Some competing traditions in experiential learning. In *Making Sense of Experiential Learning: Diversity in Theory and Practice:* S.W. Warner Weil, I. McGill eds.: Milton Keynes: Open University Press.

Brookfield S. (1987). *Developing Critical Thinkers: Challenging Adults to Explore Alternative Ways of Thinking and Acting:* Milton Keynes: Open University Press.

Brown R. (1965). *Social Psychology,* London: Collier Macmillan.

Buber M. (1958). *I and Thou:* New York: Scribener.

Buber M. (1965). *The Knowledge of Man:* New York: Harper and Row.

Burnard P. (1987). *A Study of the Ways In Which Experiential Learning Methods Are Used to Develop Interpersonal Skills in Nurses in Canada and the USA*, London: Florence Nightingale Memorial Committee.

Burnard P. (1989). *Counselling Skills for Health Professionals*, London: Chapman and Hall.

Burnard P. (1988). Preventing burnout, *Journal of District Nursing*, **7**, 5, 1988.

Burnard P. (1989B). *Teaching Interpersonal Skills: A Handbook of Experiential Learning for Health Professionals*, London: Chapman and Hall.

Burnard P. (1989c). *Exploring nurse educators' views of experiential learning*, *Nurse Education Today*, **9**, 39-45.

Burnard P., Morrison P. (1988). Nurses' perceptions of their interpersonal skills: a descriptive study using six category intervention analysis; *Nurse Education Today*, **8**, 266-272.

Campbell A. (1984). *Moderated Love*, London: SPCK.

Canfield, J., Wells H.C. (1976). *100 Ways to Enhance Self Concept in the Classroom*, New Jersey: Prentice Hall.

Claus K.E., Bailey J.T. (1980). *Living With Stress and Promoting Well Being: a Handbook for Nurses:* St Louis, Missouri: CV Mosby.

Claxton, G. (1984). *Live and Learn: an Introduction to the Psychology of Growth and Change in Everyday Life:* London: Harper and Row.

Cox M. (1978). *Structuring the Therapeutic Process*, Oxford: Pergamon.

Dass R. (1977). *The Only Dance There Is*, New York: Anchor Press.

Devine E.C., Cook T.D. (1983). A meta-analytical analysis of effects of psychoeducational interventions on length of postsurgical hospital stay, *Nursing Research* **32**, **5**, 267-274.

Dewey J., (1958). *Experience and Nature*. New York: Dover.

Dewey J., (1966). *Democracy and Education*. New York: The Free Press, Macmillan.

Dewey J., (1971). *Experience and Education*, New York: Collier Macmillan.

Egan G. (1982). *The Skilled Helper: Models, Skills and Methods for Effective Helping:* 2nd edn, Monterey: Brooks/Cole.

Eliot T.S. (1963). Collected Poems 1909-1962 London: Faber.

Ellis, R., Whittington D. (1981). *A Guide to Social Skills Training*, London: Croom Helm.

Engstrom B. (1984). The patient's need for information during hospital stay, *International Journal of Nursing Studies*, **21**, 113-130.

Feldenkrais M. (1972). *Awareness Through Movement*, New York: Harper and Row.

Freire P. (1970). *Cultural Action for Freedom*, Harmondsworth, Penguin.

Freire P. (1972). *Pedagogy of the Oppressed*, Harmondsworth: Penguin.

Freire P. (1985). *The Politics of Education*, South Hadley, Mass: Bergin and Garvey.

Freire P. (1986). Keynote Address. Presented at Workshop on Worker Education, City College of New York Center for Worker Education, New York, Feb 8th 1986.

Fromm E. (1975). *The Art of Loving:* London: Allen and Unwin.

Fromm E. (1979). *To Have or To Be?* London: Abacus.

Gale D. (1989). Moreno's approach to humanistic psychology: self and society, *The European Journal of Humanistic Psychology,* **17, 7,** 9–14.

Glasser B., Strauss A.L. (1967) *The Discovery of Grounded Theory,* Chicago: Aldine.

Gray H. (1986). Experiential learning with adults: self and society, *European Journal of Humanistic Psychology,* **4, 6,** 282–286.

Hargie O., Saunders C., Dickson D. (1987) *Social Skills in Interpersonal Communication,* London: Croom Helm.

Hayward J. (1975). *Information: A Prescription Against Pain,* London: RCN.

Heron J. (1970). *The Phenomenology of the Gaze,* Guildford: Human Potential Research Project, University of Surrey.

Heron J. (1973). *Experiential Training Techniques,* Guildford, Human Potential Research Project, University of Surrey.

Heron J. (1974b). Oepn letter to Harvey Jackins: self and society, *European Journal of Humanistic Psychology,* No 5.

Heron J. (1977). *Catharsis in Human Development,* Guildford: Human Potential Research Project, University of Surrey.

Heron J. (1977b). *Behaviour Analysis in Education and Training, Guildford: Human Potential Research Project, University of Surrey.*

Heron J. (1977c). *Dimension of Facilitator Style: Human Potential Research Project,* Guildford: University of Surrey.

Heron J. (1978). *Co-Counselling Teacher's Manual,* Guildford: Human Potential Research Project, University of Surrey.

Heron J. (1981). Philosophical basis for a new paradigm. In *Human Inquiry: A Sourcebook of New Paradigm Research,* (P. Reason, J. Rowan eds., Chichester: Wiley.

Heron J. (1986). *Six Category Intervention Analysis,* 2nd Edn, Guildford: Human Potential Research Project, University of Surrey

Heron J. (1989a). *Six Category Intervention Analysis,* 3rd edn, Guildford: Human Potential Resource Group, University of Surrey.

Heron J. (1989b). *The Facilitators' Handbook,* London: Kogan Page.

Heron J., Reason P. (1981). *Co-Counselling: an Experiential Inquiry I,* Guildford: University of Surrey, Human Potential Resource Group.

Heron J., Reason P. (1982). *Co-Counselling: an Experiential Inquiry II,* Guildford: University of Surrey, Human Potential Resource Group.

Hewitt J. (1978). *Meditation,* Sevenoaks: Hodder and Stoughton.

Illich I. (1973). *Deschooling Society,* Harmondsworth: Penguin.

Jackins H. (1965). *The Human Side of Human Beings,* Seattle: Ration Island Publishers.

Jackins H. (1970). *Fundamentals of Co-counselling Manual,* Seattle: Rational Island Publishers.

Jarvis P. (1983). *The Theory and Practice of Adult and Continuing Education,* London: Croom Helm.

Jarvis P. (1984). *The Sociology of Adult and Continuing Education*, London: Croom Helm.

Jourard S. (1964). *The Transparent Self*, New York: Van Nostrand.

Jung C.G. (1938). Psychology and Religion. In *Collected Works* Vol. 2. London: Routledge and Kegan Paul.

Jung C.G. (1978). *Man and His Symbols*, London: Picador.

Kagan C.M. (ed) (1985). *Interpersonal Skills In Nursing: Research and Applications*, Croom Helm: London.

Kagan C., Evans, J., Kay B. (1986). *A Manual of Interpersonal Skills for Nurses: an Experiential Approach*, London: Harper and Row.

Kelly G. (1955). *The Psychology of Personal Constructs* Vols I and II, New York: Norton.

Kenworthy N., Nicklin P. (1989). *Teaching and Assessing in Nursing Practice: an Experiential Approach*, London: Scutari.

Kilty, J. (1982). *Experiential Learning*, Guildford: Human Potential Research Project, University of Surrey.

Kirschenbaum, H. (1979). *On Becoming Carl Rogers*, New York: Dell.

Knowles M. (1980). *The Modern Theory and Practice of Adult Education*, Chicago: Follett.

Knowles M. (1984). *Andragogy in Action: Applying Modern Principles of Adult Learning*, San Francisco: Jossey Bass.

Knowles M. (1978). *The Adult Learner: a Neglected Species*, 2nd edn, Houston, Texas: Gulf.

Knowles M. (1975). *Self-Directed Learning*, New York: Cambridge Books.

Koberg D., Bagnall D. (1981). *The Revised All New Universal Traveller: a Soft-Systems Guide to Creativity and Problem Solving and The Process of Reaching Goals*, Los Altos, California: Kaufmann.

Kolb D. (1984). *Experiential Learning*, New Jersey: Prentice Hall.

Laing R.D. (1959). *The Divided Self*, Harmondsworth: Penguin.

Lawrence, Brother (1981). *The Practice of the Presence of God*, Sevenoaks: Hodder and Stoughton.

Le Shan L. (1974). *How to Meditate*, Wellingborough: Turnstone Press.

Lee H. (1960). *To Kill a Mockingbird*, Heinemann: London.

Lewin K. (1952). *Field Theory and Social Change*, London: Tavistock.

Lowen A. (1967). *The Betrayal of the Body*, New York: Macmillan.

Luft J. (1967). *Of Human Interaction: The Johari Model*, Palo Alto, California: Mayfield.

Mahrer A.L. (1989). A case of fundamentally different existential-humanistic psychologies, *Journal of Humanistic Psychology*, **29, 2,** 249-261.

Maslach C. (1981). *Burnout: The Cost of Caring*, New Jersey: Prentice Hall.

Maslow, A. (1972). *Motivation and Personality:* 2nd edn, New York: Harper and Row.

May R. (1989). Answer to Ken Wilber and John Rowan, *Journal of Humanistic Psychology*, **29, 2,** 244-248.

McIntee J., Firth H. (1984). How to Beat the Burnout, *Health and Social Services Journal*, 9th Feb, 166-8.

Miles R. (1987). Experiential learning in the classroom. In *The Curriculum in Nursing Education*, (P. Allan, M. Jolley eds.): Croom Helm, London.

Moreno J.L. (1959). *Psychodrama Vol 2*, Beacon, New York: Beacon House Press.

Moreno J.L. (1969). *Psychodrama Vol 3*, Beacon, New York: Beacon House Press.

Moreno J.L. (1977) *Psychodrama Vol 1:* 4th Edn, Beacon, New York: Beacon House Press.

Morrison P., Burnard P. (1989). Students' and trained nurses' perceptions of their own interpersonal skills: a report and comparison, *Journal of Advanced Nursing*, **14**, 321-329.

Morrison P. (1989). Nursing and caring: a personal construct theory study of some nurses' self-perceptions, *Journal of Advanced Nursing*, **14**, 421-426.

Moustakas C. (1984). *Finding Yourself, Finding Others*, Englewood Cliffs, New Jersey: Prentice Hall.

Nelson-Jones R. (1981). *The Theory and Practice of Counselling Psychology*, London: Holt Rinehart and Winston.

Ornstein R.E. (1975). *The Psychology of Consciousness*, Harmondsworth: Penguin.

Pearce J.C. (1982). *The Bond of Power: Meditation and Wholeness*, London: Routledge.

Perls F. (1969a). *Ego, Hunger and Aggression*, New York: Random House.

Perls F. (1969b). *Gestalt Therapy Verbatim*, Lafayette, California: Real People Press.

Peters R.S. (1972). Education as initiation. In *Philosophical Analysis and Education*, (R.D. Archambault ed.): London: Routledge and Kegan Paul.

Petty J. (1962) *Apples of Gold*, New York: Walker and Co.

Pfeiffer J.W,. Jones J.E. (1974). *A Handbook of Structured Experiences for Human Relations Training*, La Jolla, California: University Associates.

Polanyi M. (1958) *Personal Knowledge*, Chicago: University of Chicago Press.

Pring R. (1976). *Knowledge and Schooling*, London: Open Books.

Progoff I. (1985). *The Dynamics of Hope*, New York: Dialogue House Library.

Reason P., Rowan J. (1981). *Human Inquiry: a Sourcebook of New Paradigm Research*, Chichester: Wiley.

Reich. W. (1949). *Character Analysis*, New York: Simon and Schuster.

Reyner J.H. (1984). *The Gurdjieff Inheritance*, Wellingborough: Turnstone Press.

Rogers C.R. (1952). *Client-Centred Therapy*, London: Constable.

Rogers C.R. (1967). *On Becoming a Person*, London: Constable.

Rogers C.R. (1972). The process of the basic encounter group, In *Group Procedures: Purposes, Processes and Outcomes*, (R. Dietrich, H.H.H.A Dye eds.) Boston, Mass: Houghton Mifflin.

Rogers C.R. (1983). *Freedom to Learn for the Eighties*, Columbus, Ohio: Merrill.

Rogers C.R. (1985). Towards a More Human Science of the Person, *Journal of Humanistic Psychology*, **25**, 7-24.

Rogers, C.R., Stevens B. (1967). *Person to Person: The Problem of Being Human*, Lafayette, California: Real People Press.

Rolf I. (1973). *Structural Integration*, New York: Viking Press.

Rowan J. (1988). *Ordinary Ecstasy: Humanistic Psychology in Action*, London: Routledge.

Rowan J. (1989). Two humanistic psychologies or one? *Journal of Humanistic Psychology*, **29, 2,** 224-229.

Rowan J. (1989). The self: one or many?, *The Psychologist, Bulletin of the British Psychological Society*, **7,** 279-281.

Ryle, G. (1949). *The Concept of Mind*, Harmondsworth: Peregrine.

Sartre J.P. (1956). *Being and Nothingness*, New York: Philosophical Library.

Sartre J.P. (1973). *Humanism and Existentialism*, London: Methuen.

Sathe V. (1983). Implications of Corporate Culture: A Manager's Guide to Action, *Organisational Dynamics*, **12,** 5-23.

Schutz W. (1973). *Elements of Encounter*, New York: Irvington.

Searle J.R. (1983). *Intentionality: an Essay in Philosophy of Mind*, Cambridge: Cambridge University Press.

Shafer J.B.P. (1978). *Humanistic Psychology*, New Jersey: Prentice Hall.

Shor I. (1980). *Critical Teaching and Everyday Life*, Boston Mass: South End Press.

Schulman E.D. (1982). *Intervention in Human Services: A Guide to Skills and Knowledge*, 3rd Edn, St Louis, Toronto: C.V. Mosby.

Simon S.B., Howe L.W., Kirschenbaum H. (1978). *Values Clarification*, revised edition, New York: A and W Visual Library.

Singer P. (1980). *Marx*, Oxford: Oxford University Press.

Smith P.B. (1980). *Group Processes and Personal Change*, London: Harper and Row.

Spinelli E. (1989). *The Interpreted World: an Introduction to Phenomenological Psychology*, London, Sage.

Spolin V. (1963). Improvizations for the Theatre, Evanston, Illinois: Northwestern University Press.

Steel S.M., Harmon V.M. (1983). *Values Clarification in Nursing*, 2nd edn, Norwalk, C.O.: Appleton-Century-Crofts.

Stevens J.O. (1971). *Awareness: Exploring, Experimenting, Experiencing*, Moab, Utah: Real People Press.

Tart C. ed. (1969). *Altered States of Consciousness*, New York: Wiley.

Tomlinson A. (1985). The use of experiential methods in teaching interpersonal skills to nurses. In *Interpersonal Skills in Nursing: Research and Applications*, (C.M. Kagan ed.) London: Croom Helm.

Totton N., Edmonston E. (1988). *Reichian Growth Work: Melting Blocks to Life and Love*, Bridport, Prism Press.

Tuckman B.W. (1965). Developmental sequences in small groups, *Psychological Bulletin* **63, 6,** 384-99.

Vaughan F. (1984). Discovering transpersonal identity, *Journal of Humanistic Psychology,* **25, 3,** 13-38.

Vonnegut K. (1968). *Mother Night,* London: Cape.

Walker D. S. (1987). *Using Groups to Help People,* London: Routledge.

Weill S. (1967). *Waiting on God,* London: Fontana.

Whitehead A.N. (1932). *The Aims of Education,* London: Benn.

Wilber K. (1983). *Up From Eden: a Transpersonal View of Human Evolution,* London: Routledge.

Wilber K. (1989). Two humanistic psychologies or one? A response, *Journal of Humanistic Psychology,* **29, 2,** 230-243.

Woolfolk R.L., Sass L.A. (1989). Behaviourism and existentialism revisted, *Journal of Humanistic Psychology,* **28, 1,** 108-119.

Zahourek R.P. ed. (1988). *Relaxation and Imagery: Tools for Therapeutic Communication and Intervention,* Philadelphia, PA: Saunders.

Zweig F. (1965). *The Quest for Fellowship,* Oxford: Heinemann.

BIBLIOGRAPHY

Abrami P., Leenthal L., Perry R. (1982). Educational seduction, *Review of Educational Research*, **52,** 446-464.

Adler R., Rosenfeld L., Towne N. (1986). *Interplay: The Process of Interpersonal Communication, 3rd edn., New York: Holt Rinehart and Winston.*

Argyris C. (1982). *Reasoning, Learning and Action, San Franciso: Jossey Bass.*

Argyris C., Schon D. (1974). *Theory in Practice: Increasing Professional Effectiveness,* San Francisco: Jossey Bass.

Arnold E., Boggs K. (1989). *Interpersonal Relationships: Professional Communication Skills for Nurses,* Philadelphia, P.A.: Saunders.

Bailey R. (1985). *Coping With Stress in Caring,* Oxford: Blackwell.

Bailey R., Clarke M. (1989). *Stress and Coping in Nursing,* London: Chapman and Hall

Baruth L.G. (1987). *An Introduction to the Counselling Profession,* Englewood Cliffs, New Jersey: Prentice Hall.

Belkin G.S. (1984). *Introduction to Counselling,* Dubuque, Iowa: Brown.

Blackham C. (1969). *Humanism,* Harmondsworth: Pelican.

Bolger A.W. ed. (1982). *Counselling in Britain, London: Batsford Academic.*

Boone E.J., Shearon R.W., White E.E. and Associates (1980). *Serving Personal and Community Needs Through Adult Education,* San Francisco, California: Jossey Bass.

Boot R., Reynolds M. (1983). *Learning and Experience in Formal Education, Manchester: Manchester Monograph, Department of Adult and Higher Education.*

Boshier R. (1980). *Towards a Learning Society,* Vancouver, Canada: Learning Press.

Boud D., Prosser M.T. (1980). Sharing responsibility: staff-student co-operation in learning, *British Journal of Educational Technology,* **II, 1:** 24-35.

Boud D., Keogh R., Walker M. (1985). *Reflection: Turning Experience into Learning, London: Kogan Page.*

Bower G.H., Hilgard E.R. (1981). *Theories of Learning,* 5th edn, Englewood Cliffs, New Jersey: Prentice Hall.

Boydel T. (1976). *Experiential Learning: Manchester Monograph No 5, Manchester: Department of Adult and Higher Education, University of Manchester.*

Boydel E.M., Fales A.W. (1983). Reflective learning: key to learning from experience, Journal of Humanistic Psychology, **23, 2,** 99-117.

Brandes D., Phillips R. (1984). *The Gamester's Handbook, Vol 2, London: Hutchinson.*

226 *Learning Human Skills*

Brocket R., Hiemstra R. (1985). Bridging the theory-practice gap in self-directed learning, In *New Directions for Continuing Education* No 25, San Francisco, California: Jossey Bass.

Brown D., Srebalus D.J. (1988). *An Introduction to the Counselling Process:* Philadelphia, PA: Prentice Hall.

Brown I.B. ed. (1975). *The Live Classroom*, California: Esalen/Viking.

Brown S.D., Lent R.W. eds. (1984). *Handbook of Counselling Psychology: Chichester: Wiley.*

Brundage D.H., Mackeracher D. (1980). *Adult Learning Principles and their Application to Program Planning*, Ontario: Ministry of Education.

Burnard P. (1985). The Teacher as Facilitator: *Senior Nurse*, **3, 1,** 34-37.

Burnard P. (1987). Spiritual distress and the nursing response, *Journal of Advanced Nursing*, **12,** 377-382.

Burnard P. (1987). Self and peer assessment, *Senior Nurse*, **6, 5,** 16-17.

Burnard P. (1988). The Heart of the Counselling Relationship, *Senior Nurse*, **8, 12,** 17-18.

Burnard P. (1988). Coping with other people's emotions, *The Professional Nurse*, **4, 1,** 11-14.

Burnard P. (1988). Stress and relaxation in health visiting: *Health Visitor*, **61, 9,** 272.

Burnard P. (1989). Role-play, *Journal of District Nursing*, **7, 11,** 16-17.

Burnard P., Chapman C.M. (1988). *Professional and Ethical Issues in Nursing: The Code of Professional Conduct*, Chichester: Wiley.

Calnan J. (1983). *Talking With Patients*, Oxford: Heinemann.

Campbell A.V. (1981). *Rediscovering Pastoral Care*, Longman and Todd, London: Darton.

Campbell A. (1984). *Paid to Care?:* London: S.P.C.K.

Carkuff R.R. (1969). *Helping and Human Relations: Vol I: Selection and Training*, New York: Holt, Rinehart and Winston.

Chene A. (1983). The concept of autonomy in adult education, *Adult Education Quarterly*, **32, 1,** 38-47.

Clift J.C., Imrie B.W. (1981). *Assessing Students and Appraising Teaching*, London, Croom Helm.

Coleman J.S. (1982). Experiential learning and information assimilation, *Child and Youth Servises*, **14,** 3-4, 12-20.

Conrad D., Hedin D. (1982). The Impact of Experiential Education on Adolescent Development, *Child and Youth Services*, **4,** 3-4, 57-76.

Corey F. (1983). *I Never Knew I Had A Choice*, 2nd edn. California: Brooks-Cole.

Cormier L.S. (1987). *The Professional Counsellor: a Process Guide to Helping*, Englewood Cliffs, New Jersey: Prentice Hall.

Cross K.P. (1981). Adults as Learners, San Francisco: Jossey Bass.

Cross-Durrant A. (1984). Lifelong education in the writings of John Dewey, *International Journal of Lifelong Education*, **3, 2,** 115-125.

Davis C.M. (1981). Affective Education for the health Professions, *Physical Therapy*, **61, 11,** 1587-1593.

Davis B.D. ed. (1983) *Research into Nurse Education*, London: Croom Helm.

Davis B ed. (1987). *Nursing education: Research and Developments*, London: Croom Helm.

Dixon D.N., Glover J.A. (1984). *Counselling: a problem solving approach*, Chichester: Wiley.

Dowd C. (1983). Learning through experience, *Nursing Times*, 27th July, 50-52.

Dowrick P., Briggs S.J. eds. (1983). *Using Video: Psychological and Social Applications, New York: Wiley*.

Edelstein B., Eisler R. (1976). Effects of modelling and modelling with instruction and feedback, *Behaviour Therapy*, **4,** 382-389.

Edmunds M. (1983). The nurse preceptor role, *Nurse Practitioner*, **8, 6,** 52-53.

Egan G. (1986). *Exercises in Helping Skills*, 3rd edn. Monterey, California: Brooks/Cole.

Elias J.L., Merriam S. (1980). *Philosophical Foundations of Adult Education, Florida: Krieger.*

Ernst S., Goodison L. (1981). *In our Own Hands: a Book of Self Help Therapy*, London: The Womens' Press.

Famighetti R.A. (1981). Experiential Learning: The close encounters of the institutional kind, *Gerontology and Geriatric Education*, **2, 2,** 129-132.

Ferruci P. (1982). *What We May Be, Wellingborough: Turnstone Press.*

Flyn P.A.R. (1980). *Holistic Health: The Art and Science of Care, Bowie, Maryland: Brady.*

Fox F.E. (1983). The spiritual core of experiential education, *Journal of Experiential Education*, **16, 1,** 3-6.

Frankl V.E. (1959). *Mans Search for Meaning*, New York: Beacon Press.

Frankl V.E. (1978). *The Unheard Cry for Meaning*, New york: Simon and Schuster.

Gager R. (1982). Experiential Education: Strengthening the Learning Process, *Child and Youth Services*, **4, 3 ⟩ 4,** 31-39.

Geller L. (1985). Another look at self-actualization *Journal of Humanistic Psychology*, **24, 2,** 93-106

Gerard B., Boniface W., Love B. (1980). *Interpersonal Skills for Health Professionals, Reston, V.A.: Reston Publishing Co.*

Gibson R.L., Mitchell M.H. (1986). *Introduction to Counselling and Guidance*, London: Collier Macmillan.

Gorden D. (1982). The concept of the hidden curriculum, *Journal of Philosophy of Education*, **16, 2,** 187-188.

Gross R. (1977). *The Lifelong Learner*, New York: Simon and Schuster.

Grossman R. (1985). Some Reflections on Abraham Maslow, *Journal of Humanistic Psychology*, **25, 4,** 31-34.

228   *Learning Human Skills*

Halmos P. (1965). *The Faith of the Counsellors*, London: Constable.

Hamilton M.S. (1981). Mentorhood: a key to nursing leadership, *Nursing Leadership*, **4, 1,** 4-13.

Hanks L., Belliston L., Edwards D. (1977). *Design Yourself, Los Altos, California: Kaufman.*

Hare A.P. (1976). *Handbook of Small Group Research,* New York: Free Press.

Harris T. (1969). *I'm O.K., Your O.K.,* London: Harper and Row.

Hendricks G., Fadiman J. eds. (1976). *Transpersonal Education: a Curriculum for Feeling and Being,* Englewood Cliffs, New Jersey: Prentice Hall.

Hendricks G., Weinhod B. (1982). Transpersonal Approaches to Counselling and Psychotherapy, Denver, Colorado: Love Publishing Co.

Herinck R. ed. (1980). *The Psychotherapy Handbook,* New York: New American Library.

Hinchliff S. M. ed (1979). *Teaching in Clinical Nursing,* Edinburgh: Churchill Livingstone.

Holt R. (1982). An alternative to mentorship, *Adult Education,* **55, 2,** 152-156.

Houle C.O. (1984). *Patterns of Learning,* San Francisco: Jossey Bass.

Hurding R.F. (1985). *Roots and Shoots: a Guide to Counselling and Psychotherapy,* London: Hodder and Stoughton.

Hutchins D.E. (1987). *Helping Relationships and Strategies,* Monterey, California: Brooks-Cole.

Ivey A.E. (1987). *Counselling and Psychotherapy: Skills, theories and practice,* London: Prentice Hall International.

James M., Jongeward D. (1971). *Born to Win: Transactional Analysis With Gestalt Experiments,* Reading, Mass: Addison-Wesley.

Jarvis P. (1983). *Professional Education,* London: Croom Helm.

Jarvis P. (1987). Meaningful and meaningless experience: towards an understanding, Adult Education Quarterly, **37, 3.**

Jenkins E. (1987). *Facilitating Self-Awareness: a Learning Package Combining Group,* Wigan: Open Software Library.

Jourard S. (1971). *Self-Disclosure: an Experimental Analysis of the Transparent Self,* New York: Wiley.

Jung C.G. (1976). *Modern Man in Search of a Soul,* London: Routledge and Kegan Paul.

Kelly G.A. (1970). A brief introduction to personal construct theory, In (Bannister, D. ed.: *Perspectives in Construct Theory,* London: Academic Press.

Kennedy E. (1979). *On Becoming a Counsellor,* London: Gill and Macmillan.

Kilty J. (1978). *Self and Peer Assessment,* Guildford: Human Potential Research Project, University of Surrey.

Kilty J. (1987). *Staff Development for Nurse Education: Practitioners Supporting Staff,* Guildford, Surrey: Human Potential Research Project: University of Surrey.

King E.C. (1984). *Affective Education in Nursing*, A Guide to Teaching and Assessment, Maryland: Aspen.

Knox A.B. ed (1980). *Teaching Adults Effectively*, San Francisco, California: Jossey Bass.

Kottler J.A., Brown R.W. (1985). *Introduction to Therapeutic Counselling*, Monterey, California: Brooks-Cole.

Legge D. (1982). *The Education of Adults In Britain*, Milton Keynes: Open University Press.

Levine A. (1985). The Pollyana Paradigm, *Journal of Humanistic Psychology*, **25, I,** 90–93

Levison R.H. (1979). Experiential Education Abroad, *Teaching Sociology*, **6, 4,** 415–419.

Lipsett L., Avakian N.A. (1981). Assessing experiential learning: lifelong learning, *The Adult Years*, **5, 2,** 18–22.

Lowen A., Lowen L. (1977). *The Way to Vibrant Health: A Manual of Bioenergetic Exercises*, New York: Harper and Row.

Maple F.F. (1985). *Dynamic Interviewing: An Introduction to Counselling*, Beverly Hills, California: Sage.

Marshall L.A., Rowland F. (1983). *A Guide to Learning Independently*, Milton Keynes: Open University Press.

McPeck J.E. (1981). *Critical Thinking and Education*, New York: St. Martins Press.

Menson B. ed. (1982). *Building on Experiences in Adult Development: New Directions for Experiential Learning No 16*, San Francisco, California: Jossey Bass.

Merriam S. (1984). Mentors and Proteges: a Critical Review of the Literature, *Adult Education Quarterly*, **33, 3,** 161–173.

Mezeiro J. (1981). A critical theory of adult learning and education, *Adult Education*, **32, I,** 3–24.

Mocker D.W., Spear G.E. (1982). *Lifelong Learning: Formal, Non-formal and Self-Directed*, Columbus, Ohio: The ERIC Clearinghouse on Adult Career and Vocational Education.

Morsund J. (1985). *The Process of Counselling and Therapy:* Englewood Cliffs, New Jersey: Prentice Hall.

Murgatroyd S., Woolfe R. (1982). *Coping with Crisis-Understanding and Helping Persons in Need*, London: Harper and Row.

Murgatroyd S. (1986). Counselling and Helping, *British Psychological Society*, London: Methuen.

Myerscough P.R. (1989). *Talking With Patients: A Basic Clinical Skill*, Oxford: Oxford Medical Publications.

Nadler L. ed (1984). *The Handbook of Human Resource Development*, New York: Wiley.

Naranjo C., Ornstein R.E. (1971). *On the Psychology of Meditation*, London: Allen and Unwin.

Nelson-Jones R. (1984). *Personal Responsibility: counselling and therapy: an integrative approach.*, London: Harper and Row.

Nelson-Jones R. (1988). *Practical Counselling and Helping Skills: helping clients to help*, London: Cassell.

Noble P. (1983). *Formation of Freirian Facilitators*, Chicago: Latino Institute.

Nyberg D. ed (1975). *The Philosophy of Open Education*, London: Routledge and Kegan Paul.

Ohlsen A.M., Horne A.M., Lawe C.F. (1988). *Group Counselling*, New York: Holt Rinehart and Winston.

Open University Coping With Crisis Group (1987). *Running Workshops: A Guide for Trainers in the Helping Professions*, London: Croom Helm.

Patton M.Q. (1982). *Practical Evaluation*, Beverly Hills, California: Sage.

Postman N., Weingartner C.W. (1969). *Teaching as a Subversive Activity*: Penguin, Harmondsworth.

Procter B. (1978). *Counselling Shop*, London: Deutsch.

Rawlings M.E., Rawlings L. (1983). Mentoring and networking for helping professionals, *Personnel and Guidance Journal*, **62, 2,** 116-118.

Reddy M. (1987). *The Manager's Guide to Counselling at Work*, London: Methuen.

Riebel L. (1984). A homeopathic model of psychotherapy, *Journal of Humanistic Psychology*, **24, 1,** 9-48.

Ringuette E.L. (1983). A note on experiential learning in professional training, *Journal of Clinical Psychology*, **39, 2,** 302-304.

Rogers C.R. (1957). The necessary and sufficient conditions of therapeutic personality change, *Journal of Consulting Psychology*, **21,** 95-104.

Rowan J. (1986). Holistic listening, *Journal of Humanistic Psychology*, **26, 1,** 83-102.

Schon D.A. (1983). *The Reflective Practitioner: How Professionals Think in Action*, New York: Basic Books.

Shapiro E.C., Haseltime F., Rowe M. (1978). *Moving up: role models, mentors and the patron system, Sloan management review*, **19,** 51-58.

Shapiro S.B. (1985). An empirical analysis of operating values in humanistic education, *Journal of Humanistic Psychology*, **25, 1,** 94-108

Shropshire C.O. (1981). Group experiential learning in adult education, *The Journal of Continuing Education in Nursing*, **12, 6,** 5-9.

Smith E.W.L. ed. (1976). *The Growing Edge of Gestalt Therapy*, Secaucus, New Jersey, Citadel Press.

Stitch T.F. (1983). Experiential Therapy, *Journal of Experiential Education*, **5, 3,** 23-30.

Tough A.M. (1982). *Intentional Changes; A Fresh Approach to Helping People Change*, New York: Cambridge Books.

Trower P. ed. (1984). *Radical Approaches to Social Skills Training*, London, Croom Helm.

Truax C.B., Carkuff R.R. (1967). *Towards Effective Counselling and Psychotherapy*, Chicago: Aldine.

Van Deurzen-Smith E (1988). *Existential Counselling in Practice*, Beverly Hills: Sage.

Wallace W.A. (1986). *Theories of Counselling and Psychotherapy: a Basic Issues Approach:* Boston: Allyn and Bacon.

Wheeler D.D., Janis I.L. (1980). *A Practical Guide for Making Decisions,* New York: Free Press.

Wlodkowski R.J. (1985). *Enhancing Adult Motivation to Learn,* San Francisco, California: Jossey Bass.

INDEX OF
EXERCISES

Counselling Exercises

INDEX

Action in experiential learning 40–1
Aims of experiential learning activities
    77, 81, 82, *see also specific
    exercises*
America, North, experiential learning
    in 71–3
Andragogy and experiential learning
    64–7
Anger 133
Appearance, developing awareness of
    one's 26
Assessment *see* Evaluation
Attending (paying/giving attention):
    in counselling 98–112
        exercises 107–11
    in groups, exercises 162–3
Attention 22–4
    on fantasy 23–4
    focused in 22–4
    focused out 22, 23
        exercises in getting 99–100
    paying/giving *see* Attending
Authentic person 3–4
Authoritative interventions 113
Awareness:
    body- *see* Body
    exercises in 84
    self- *see* Self-awareness

Behaviour 9–10
    interpreting 20–1
Blind walking, exercise of 174
Body, experience of the
    (body-awareness) 17–19, 28
    exercises exploring 211–13
Bodywork methods 18–19, 28
Brain-storming 58
Breaths, counting the 207
Buber, M. 4, 90
'Burnout' in nurses 59

Carers, complusive 156
Catalytic interventions 113, 116, 117,
    138–44
    examples 139
    exercises 138–44
Catharsis *see* Emotions
Cathartic interventions 113, 116, 117,
    133–8
    examples 135
    exercises 136–8
Cathartic style of facilitation 180,
    190–1
    exercises in 190–1
Client:
    counsellor and, taking turns to be,
        in co-counselling 48–51
    rate of development of relationship
        with counsellor determined by
        98
Client-centred counselling 46
Closing a group, exercises on 179
Co-counselling 48–51
Cohesiveness, group, exercise
    exploring 177–8
Complimenting exercises 84
Confronting interventions 113, 116,
    117, 129–32
    exercises 129–32
Confronting style of facilitation 180,
    189
    exercises in 189
Consciousness, self- 19–20
Conversational ability of nurse
    teachers, informal 36–7
Counselling 89–148
    client-centred 46
    co- 48–51
    interventions *see* Interventions
    processes 96–8
    skills: